HOMOEOPATHY IN EPIDEMIC DISEASES

T0333129

HOMOEOPATHY
IN
EPIDEMIC DISEASES

by

Dr. DOROTHY SHEPHERD

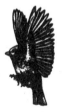

THE C.W. DANIEL COMPANY LIMITED

1 Church Path, Saffron Walden, Essex, England

First published 1967

Reprinted 1981

Reprinted (in paperback) 1996, 2010

12

© Mrs. G. E. Robinson 1967

ISBN 978 0 852 07305 6

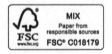
Printed and bound in Great Britain by Clays Ltd, Elcograf S.p.A.

CONTENTS

FOREWORD

AMONG the many books written on Homoeopathy, there has not been one on epidemic diseases which would be of interest to the lay reader, or inspire an enquirer with zest for further information regarding the Homoeopathic approach to health and disease. This fact was of much concern to the late Dr. Dorothy Shepherd, for she had great sympathy at all times with those who were striving to use Homoeopathy sensibly in their daily living when the need arose.

She was a busy doctor, much sought after for her advice and help; always ready and willing to share her thoughts and knowledge on the subject which, before everything else, absorbed her life. Yet she felt there were many who, knowing little or nothing of this vast study of Homoeopathic Principle, could benefit by having books simply written in easily understood terms on the everyday illnesses which could sweep through a nation or a country.

Epidemic diseases could so often, in her opinion, have been halted by the correct Homoeopathic remedy administered at the first indication of disorder—the one time of supreme importance in the control of epidemics. Even the layman, if well informed, could take or give, with safety, the indicated remedy, and then refer to the qualified doctor for subsequent help. With this in mind, she began to write short chapters on the most generally known epidemic disorders—whether she would have expanded them later, I do not know.

I have collected together all Dorothy Shepherd's

writings relating to these various diseases and know that in presenting them to the public, another valuable contribution will have been added to the knowledge of those who practise this great Art of Medication. They may also provide further enlightenment and encouragement to those who are seeking an alternative approach to health and well being, for although infectious diseases are notifiable to the authorities, a dose of the correct Homœopathic remedy will shorten the duration of the illness and prevent unhappy after effects.

GWENETH E. ROBINSON

Thornbury
North Devon

EPIDEMICS

EPIDEMICS are widespread outbreaks of a disease affecting simultaneously a number of people in one or several neighbourhoods, and even whole districts, states, or countries. The character of such epidemics varies from time to time; each outbreak may be totally different from the preceding or succeeding ones, even though pathologically it may be diagnosed as the same disease, viz.—smallpox, malaria or influenza. The symptoms characterising each epidemic depend on various factors: climate, prevailing weather conditions, barometric changes, and the association of certain anopheles (mosquitoes) and swampy ground producing malaria; fleas and rats in the plague; lice for the spread of typhus—and the reactions of the individual affected towards them.

Epidemics killing whole populations have ravaged our globe for thousands of years. They were considered "visitations of the Deity", and as such had to be endured. The only sacrifices to be made by the suffering populace were of a financial nature as offerings to the priesthood, in the hope that the wrath of the Godhead might be appeased and that the evil would thereby be staved off. History is full of such incidents; the rise and fall of successive nations is frequently closely connected with epidemics raging and destroying whole tribes from antiquity to modern times. What a vast difference such epidemics have made to the progress and retrogression of successive civilisations of mankind.

Consider, for example, Greece, in its classic days of the fifth century B.C. It was a nation of most highly gifted and talented individuals. Plato, whose writings, metaphysical, philosophical and psychological are still being studied with benefit in our own day; the highly developed drama expressed in the tragedies of Aeschylus and Sophocles, still fill us with horror and pity; Pythagoras the great mathematician who taught hundreds of pupils the science of numbers and geometry and the occult wisdom based on it; architecture and sculpture had never before been expressed in such beauty or perfection and still remains in the ruins of the Acropolis at Athens to awe and inspire us. Throngs of enquiring youths from countries far and near frequented the training colleges for occult learning such as we have never yet emulated. One of the greatest physicians of all time lived in that classical age— Hippocrates, the Father of Medicine—who, trained in the temple mysteries, yet came forth to teach the principle of the curative simile, the relationship between disease and the like drug. Greek dances reached a stage approaching perfection, music was taught—who has not heard of the story of men and women and even animals listening entranced by the sweet strains which came from Orpheus and his lute, even the Spirits in the underworld were bewitched by it. Great epic writers, great lawyers, athletes, runners and warriors all graced this nation. Alexander the Great, who when only a youth, led the Greeks in his famous campaigns and extended his kingdom beyond the Euphrates into and over the borders of India. Yet he succumbed while yet under thirty years of age, not to battle, but to the malaria epidemic which raged for many years and brought about the downfall of this wonderful nation so that it sank into oblivion.

Later followed the Roman Empire and the era of great trading. The sailors roamed the seas of the then known world and brought back the treasures and luxuries of far countries to Rome. The cohorts of Roman soldiers conquered vast territories and to be made "a Roman citizen" was the greatest privilege that could be bestowed on anyone. Think of St. Paul, the Apostles, the Roman poets; the classics of Julius Caesar's "History of the Gallic Wars", of Ovid and Virgil; the Roman Law which is the basis still of English and American Legal Bar. The Romans seemed unconquerable. Alas, they became too luxury loving, the patricians looked down on the simple things of life, they preferred the luxuries from far off countries; quails and exotic fruits from North Africa. Wheat was brought from Britain. Yes, our country supplied Rome with corn, for agriculture in the environs of Rome was neglected. It is not clear whether the epidemic malaria came first and slew the farmers so that the soil could not be tilled, or whether the farmers were so discouraged because farming did not pay—due to the demand for cheap bread and free trade—there was an exodus to the towns and cities. However it may have been, the land became sour, over grown with weeds and all drainage neglected. Swamps developed which made a happy breeding ground for the anopheles, the mosquito which is the host of the malaria parasite, and malaria began to wage what is recorded as a continuous epidemic, and between the outbursts of malaria, there were epidemics of plague. Malaria does not always kill its victims, often it will only gradually enervate the sufferers, the blood cells become diseased and the spleen, the factory of blood cells, becomes enlarged. Anaemia, specially cerebral anaemia, makes the patient slack, lazy and stupid. Three to four hundred years of chronic malaria gradually exhausted the virile Roman people, and when the conquerors came from the north over the Alps—the Vandals and Goths, the malaria ridden populace fell an easy victim to them. The continent of Europe became the happy hunting ground of the uncivilised warrior tribes of the Teutonic German races and the dark middle ages followed when all culture, the belles arts, literature, were forgotten and the black death ruled the plains of Europe.

Wars, famines, pestilences reigned for nearly a thousand years. The death rate was extremely high, the expectation of life was short indeed, a matter of about twenty years. No time for an individual to gain either knowledge or experience. We have no idea how devastating such epidemics were. We can only faintly surmise by comparison with the modern pestilence, the pandemic, that is world wide epidemic, influenza. This affected about four hundred out of every thousand of the population and of these four hundred only two died. Four hundred in every thousand makes, in a population of one hundred and fifty millions, sixty millions sick and two hundred and forty thousand deaths. A large number you say, but bubonic plague affected 100 per cent of the population and killed from twenty to eighty out of every hundred affected, a vast difference. Few indeed were left after such a carnage.

In these later times we have learnt to control some of these epidemics, by means of quarantine and isolation of the contacts. But the enemy is not so far off really. He lurks in the breeding grounds in the Far East, in Asia, and at any moment, if the watchful eyes of the port sanitary authorities were removed owing to circumstances, he might be on us in some form or another. Think too how transport has improved, instead of weeks and months, it takes only hours almost to encircle the globe in one of our modern aeroplanes. A passenger or passengers may be landed in a few hours from India or China carrying the seeds to anybody, to any of the people he mixes with.

It behoves us to face the dangers squarely and prepare accordingly. Orthodox medicine has little to offer us, except isolation. This does well up to a point as a preventive, but once a disease is started, there is little treatment except perhaps with serums, vaccines and the nostrums of the sulphonamide class. These bring down the fever in a miraculous fashion, but the drug once let loose in the body, not only slays the invader, the bacteria, but when the germs are killed, it attacks the healthy cells, the red blood corpuscles and the lymphatic cells. There is then a battle during which the patient feels extremely ill, even though his temperature is down. The effects of the excess of sulphonamide may be and often are long lasting, and the patient dies at long last, a victim of the treatment, having had to put up with years of ill health, even though X-rays and blood tests may find very little wrong. Homoeopathy does not treat the disease, but the individual behind the disease, and in serious acute infectious diseases, in communicable epidemics, has conquered in the past and will conquer again if we follow its teachings.

There are rumours of epidemics on the Continent, diphtheria is increasing in spite, or is it because of immunisation? Germany is the most highly immunised country in the world and yet the death rate of diphtheria is rising fast. Typhus is following in the footsteps of famine and we do not know what else is before us. As Homoeopaths we should not be backward in pressing our claim of being able to cure, really CURE acute epidemic diseases.

We have in this country already small epidemics of many communicable diseases, such as measles, rubella or German measles and mumps, whooping cough and poliomyelitis, and I shall consider these in the following pages.

PROPHYLAXIS

EPIDEMIC diseases treated and nursed at home raise the problem of prophylaxis or prevention. And here again Homoeopathy offers the best solution. Believe me, it has been shown again and again that our medicines given intelligently and according to our law that "like cures like" do not only cure infectious diseases speedily and easily without the development of any complications, but they also prevent these same diseases. This is of great importance, particularly in the case of infants who have not enough stamina to stand up to an onslaught of whooping cough or measles or diphtheria, or infantile paralysis, the latest bugbear of the press.

If one can prevent these diseases until the children are over five years of age, the disease is usually not so fatal, and the children stand a better chance.

Of course, the modern methods of prevention of disease occupy much space in our medical literature, and apparently they are successful to a degree. The agents used in prophylaxis resemble crudely the medicines used in Homoeopathy, and some Homoeopathic physicians have been somewhat led astray by this similarity to the Homoeopathic principle, and recommend the present orthodox methods.

Are the inoculations against the various infectious diseases 100 per cent foolproof? Do they not in some cases lead to serum or vaccine disease? Is it not a fact that they often produce severe reactions? Indeed, they have been known to lead to fatal consequences. Have I been more unfortunate than the average Homoeopathic physician in seeing the negative or disease-producing effects of orthodox prophylaxis? Indeed I was not biased either in the beginning; I was extremely interested in prevention of such diseases as diphtheria and measles and the rest. It was a great disappointment to me to observe the frequent severe reactions in the wake of immunisation against diphtheria, and later on the uncertain effects of inoculations against measles, whooping cough, and scarlet fever.

Now some of my fears of the dangers inherent in the modern methods of inoculations have been proved to be well founded and correct. Some impartial medical observers in Australia have found that the incidence of poliomyelitis, the modern infantile paralysis, has vastly increased since whooping cough and diphtheria inoculations have become more popular, and that the incubation period of infantile paralysis corresponds closely to, and follows exactly on the correct day after the inoculation has been made. It might have been coincidence, if it had only happened in one or two cases, but unfortunately it has happened in more than 50 per cent of the cases.

At the moment doctors are advised not to immunise at the danger periods of the year, when infantile paralysis is most prevalent. Whether this is the first step in giving up the dangerous method of immunisation, one does not know.

My own personal opinion is, that inoculation with any type of serum in any of these infectious diseases is harmful and can easily and safely be replaced by a remedy or remedies, proved according to our Law of Similars that "like cures like" on healthy individuals. Nosodes or disease products of the actual disease are often most active preventives. This will sound revolutionary to many doctors, but for years I have been in the position to watch the results and after-effects, early

15

as well as late, of immunisation against diphtheria, and I have not been impressed.

For years I worked in closest contact with an immunisation clinic and had to convince the mothers of the great advantage that would ensue. It was somewhat difficult to deal with irate parents later on, when they had been told that the operation was painless, and they saw the swollen, congested arms which occasionally cropped up. And it was even more difficult when a child developed diphtheria after it had finished its course of inoculation! And as for that mother who lost her child of a fulminating attack of diphtheria within eight hours after the disease started when a certificate of safety had been issued from the clinic; I do not know how the immunising doctor got over that stile!

I was very unpopular, I remember, when the Medical Officer of Health was told about this fatality from diphtheria, and he remarked "This would not have happened, if the mother had had the child immunised", and I retorted that she had been well and truly done six months previously. I used to receive all the official publications on diphtheria immunisation from the said M.O.H. after this little contretemps, as if he was trying to shelter himself behind the official acts.

I therefore have no hesitation in stating that from my own experience and observation, the Homoeopathic preventives are much safer in use, and absolutely certain in their effects. Even should the infectious disease develop, it will be in a much milder form.

The earliest preventive used in Homoeopathy was *Belladonna*, which Hahnemann was the first to recommend and use successfully, both as a preservative from and curative in the disease, and it wiped out even the after-effects of scarlet fever, which were often as dangerous as the actual disease in the days when scarlet fever was at its peak.

Let me quote from his "Lesser Writings", where Hahnemann states that where ulceration followed scarlet fever and *Belladonna* was no longer of service, *Chamomilla* would remove all tendency to it in a few days, and the suffocating cough which might follow the disease was also removed by *Chamomilla*, particularly if accompanied by flushing of the face and horripilation of limbs and back. This recalls to my mind an incident from my childhood days, when a sister developed an abscess on her knee after scarlet fever, and was kept in isolation for weeks. The local doctor, a nice, capable man, could not suggest anything besides rest; we did not know about *Chamomilla* then; and in the end it cleared up after many weeks. I still recollect the violent storms of temper we had to deal with in the little patient; she was so unmanageable that she had to be sent to a boarding school. *Chamomilla* would have saved much trouble and anxiety to everybody, if this little precious hint of Hahnemann's had been known.

If the prevailing type of scarlet fever at the particular moment is not of the smooth order, but rough, miliary and dark, then *Ailanthus*, *Phytolacca* and *Sulphur* will protect those in contact with the disease, be it at school or at home, or even in hospital. Better still, discover the specific epidemic remedy and this will give the highest protection.

Protection against measles is usually found in *Pulsatilla* 6 or 30, nightly from the third or seventh day after contact, until after the danger of infection is past; that is on the fifteenth or sixteenth day. I have found this to answer extremely well in various nursery schools where we had to deal with toddlers under the age of five, the most susceptible and dangerous age. Before the use of this prophylactic, the rate of attendance in the first three months of the year used to drop to below ten in each of the three schools I was responsible for.

After the *Pulsatilla* was given almost as a routine, we had the full quota of attendance, with only occasional absentees. How different it would be if the knowledge of our preventives were more fully appreciated and believed in!

Morbillinum 30 has been used as a prophylactic in measles. This should be given at weekly intervals during the incubation period, with caution. I found in one school that all the children came down with a feverish attack, catarrhal symptoms, and a measley rash on the same day, after daily doses of *Morbillinum* had been given. I stuck to *Pulsatilla* after that experience.

Preventive agents against whooping cough: Dr. Grimmer found *Carbo. Vegetabilis* a reliable remedy in hundreds of cases of young children and infants. He qualifies it however by saying that in some epidemics, *Drosera* or *Cuprum Met.* may give the most certain protection.

Personally I have always used for years and years in whooping cough its own nosode, *Pertussin*, which Dr. John Clarke recommended so strongly in his monograph. *Pertussin* has given me 100 per cent protection even though it raged in a particular district; all the children on *Pertussin*, either in the 12th or 30th potency, given daily, escaped it.

I used it for years in the nurseries, in my private practice, in the medical clinic, and in hundreds of cases in various epidemics we went through, and truly it is a great remedy.

In one epidemic there were 120 children of varying ages, ranging from twelve months to fourteen years, on prophylactic doses; only one out of this number, an infant of eight months, died, the parents counteracting the action of the *Pertussin* by applying camphorated oil to the chest.

I was interested to hear of the beneficial effect of this

prophylactic in a small boarding school, where whooping cough was introduced by one of the boarders—a doctor's child, too—at the beginning of the term. *Pertussin* 30 was given night and morning to everyone, and the whole school escaped. The head of the school recalled a similar accidental introduction of whooping cough at her school some years previously, when all the children were infected; they had to import day and night nurses, and one of the children nearly died. She was grateful to Homoeopathy and to *Pertussin* for having saved the school from a similar dénouement.

HOW TO TAKE A CASE OF *ACUTE* DISEASE

A FAMILY practitioner, who alas, may soon be as dead as a Dodo, in these isles of ours, as well as a medical officer in a boarding school, should take careful, though necessarily short, notes in writing of all the symptoms of the patients he meets on his rounds. He will soon find that the symptoms in any epidemic are much the same or resemble one another in that particular epidemic.

At the beginning, the picture may not be very clear; soon, when the epidemic is in full swing, it will be found that there are but slight variations. An experienced medical man will soon be able to decide which are the principal remedies or remedy for the particular type of disease he is dealing with, whatever the name he may decide to give the epidemic—it might be called influenza, if there is no rash, or measles or scarlet fever, etc. if a rash is present, or diphtheria if the throat is affected.

It is true that the Homoeopathic physician has to make two diagnoses. First, the diagnosis of the disease, for the parents' sake in order to satisfy the demands of the Health Board, or the Medical Officer of Health or whatever the name of the public authority may be, and secondly, he has to diagnose the remedy, frequently, unless he is very experienced in the drugs, not an easy matter.

There is always a premonitory stage, sometimes longer, in almost every epidemic disease, when it is difficult to make a diagnosis and the orthodox physician is often at a loss what to prescribe. He may have to wait, until the disease declares itself. The physician practising our method, looks at the combination of symptoms, objective and subjective, and on these he prescribes the remedy. Frequently he will find that the disease turns out to be a very mild one or only faintly shows itself.

Many times in the early days of my practice, I was told that I was very lucky, none of my cases were ever very ill, or maybe I might have been told that I had made an error in my diagnosis. It is rather galling at first to somebody young and still lacking the assurance that experience gives, to be told such things. In course of time one can point out to the departing critics, that as all or nearly all the cases turn out to be either mild or at any rate recover much more rapidly than those treated in hospitals and/or by practitioners in the neighbourhood, there must be a common factor in the cases treated so successfully by the Homoeopathic physician. And that common factor is the knowledge of the action of the remedies; first tried out or proved systematically on healthy individuals, and only later, when the action of each remedy is strictly defined, used on the sick person.

And what a help such a knowledge is, what power the Homoeopathic physician wields over the common enemy to mankind, ill health.

The physician, in taking careful notes of all his acute cases—with temperatures, spots, nausea, different aches and pains—must study them carefully for a while, with the help of his favourite repertory or dictionary, and then later, looking up the two or three remedies chosen for comparison, until he is sure of the drugs or medicines most suitable for that particular type of epidemic. It takes time at first, but a young doctor has much leisure at the beginning and can lay a sound foundation for the future by taking such meticulous care in the early stages. He will find, that when he has written down all the abnormal signs and symptoms of all the epidemics he comes across for, one, two or three years, his memory improves so much, that he can carry many more remedies in his head and that the need for writing down each and all the abnormal variations ceases. He may have to do it at the beginning of each epidemic, but he will soon spot the prevailing disease types and the necessary remedies which will cure speedily and easily.

He will receive great help if he teaches all his patients what symptoms to look out for at every aberration from the normal. Parents, especially mothers, nurses and other adults responsible for children, who are usually and most frequently the victims in any epidemic, should be carefully instructed how they can best be of assistance to the doctor, to lighten his labour.

Careful observation is necessary, not needless fussy anxiety; just balanced, quiet observation on the part of any adult is required.

Look out for any mental or emotional variations from the normal, in a child or any sick person in their ken.

A naturally cheerful person may become fractious, irritable, refuse to be looked at or touched, or scream or weep at the slightest opposition; or an independent child may suddenly want to be cuddled or made a fuss of or refuse to be left alone. There may be nightmares, delirium, muttering and gnashing of teeth; restlessness, throwing off of clothes, wandering about; the dreams and ideas most prevalent during a delirious phase should be noted, they are very important. The sick person may think there are two or more persons in bed with him; and if the doctor is told about this, his advice of remedies would be limited straightway to two or three and he would be saved time and labour.

I had a pneumonia patient who thought in delirium that she was very cramped in bed and could not understand why there was another person lying by her side. I was wavering between *Bryonia* and *Phosphorous* and this statement clinched the diagnosis of the drug. *Phosphorus* brought down the temperature and the respiration in thirty-six hours and I had great difficulty in keeping the patient in bed even for a week. She felt so well and there was no relapse either and no complications followed.

There may be physical changes, which should be carefully observed. Changes in the colour, extreme dryness of skin or increased perspiration. There may be alterations in postures, lying all curled up in a heap, or always in one particular position, different from the usual.

Therefore the slightest variation from the usual or normal attitude of the patient should be observed and noted down. These abnormal signs and symptoms should neither be exaggerated nor decried, just carefully and judicially observed. I have had reports of an attack given to me on the telephone, so carefully and exactly given, that I could make up my mind there and then what the remedy was, and on getting to the patient, the disease picture was so correct that I could add nothing to it and the remedy decided upon was right and set the patient rapidly on to the road to recovery.

On the other hand, I have had people give me reports on the telephone who had been given instructions for years and yet they would never learn what to look for, what to report, and who had watched me at work and yet they were psychologically incapable of being truthful observers.

Yes, the taking of a case is very important and is more than half the battle in conquering ill health.

23

It is necessary to know and remember which are the essential points. Then again, the doctor must know and remember the common symptoms—symptoms common to that disease—and put them low down on his list for possibles.

In a feverish case, for example, you would expect the patient to be thirsty, if he is not, it cuts out a number of remedies; if he is thirsty and asks for warm drinks only, that again is peculiar and will enable the requisite remedy to be found quickly. And again, if he craves only for cold drinks and perhaps brings the drink up rapidly after it is down, then a certain remedy is the curative one.

Each symptom which is observed and noted should be carefully annotated as regards its modalities, its reaction to circumstances—does motion make a certain symptom worse or better? How does posture affect the patient? What difference does heat or cold or wet, hot or cold applications locally make to the pain, etc? The nature, the character, the direction, the time factor of the pain are all important, so also the time factor as regards the general amelioration or aggravation of any symptoms present in the patient. One patient is regularly at his worst at midnight, another is worse early evening, another in the afternoon, and so on. If the time aggravation is marked, then it becomes important in deciding which is the right remedy. This applies to any other symptoms present in a case. If there is diarrhoea, the character, consistency, odour of the stool or any accompanying symptoms must be noted. With vomiting, observe the minutest details, the colour of the tongue, variations in taste, the character and odour of the vomit.

You will find that a Homoeopathic physician takes a great interest in all the details of the case before him and will do it with every new patient presented to him.

I cannot but insist too strongly on the importance of taking a case properly, writing each case down in the early days, and comparing and contrasting the various details, looking them up in the repertory and also reading up other remedies chosen in the Materia Medica, the final arbitrator. Yes, it needs time at first, much time, but with greater experience, time will be shortened. Specially during epidemics you may have to spend a long period in the first few cases, but when you are familiar with the Typus Epidemicus, you will need a few notes to decide what remedy is necessary, an epidemic is usually covered by, at the most, three or four remedies.

What is the reward for all this labour? The satisfaction of seeing the patients recover, of lowering the mortality rate in your own immediate neighbourhood, the satisfaction to yourself of work well done. There is little need of sending patients to hospitals; as soon as a case is diagnosed, taking your own responsibility, treating and curing the cases at home, gives great joy to the true healer, the true physician. Not only is there a lowering of the death rate, there is also a lowering of the morbidity rate, a raising of the general standard of health. Less need for convalescence, less need for hospital beds. There is a shortage of nursing staff, of kitchen and domestic staffs in hospitals, if the children are nursed at home and recover rapidly without any ill after-effects, what a saving to the nation in general! And if the disease germs are not so concentrated as they are in hospital wards, there will be less danger of cross-infection, less danger of any child developing one infectious disease after another, as they are liable to do in a crowded ward.

DIPHTHERIA

THIS is a disease which has been surrounded by a veil of terror—the psychology of fear has been well applied so that doctors and lay people alike are terrified of the very name, yet septic throats, streptococci throats, quinsies and angina throats may prove just as fatal. The pathological diagnosis is of scientific interest, but does not help very much in finding the right remedy. There are some bold spirits in this and other countries who have defied the edict of the majority and have applied our Homoeopathic drugs with much better results than orthodox medical treatment, and one would only wish there were more who would be sufficiently courageous to abide by the Law of Similars in treating cases of diphtheria.

Before I suggest some of the remedies which will be found helpful in the cases to which they apply, I must say a few words on *Diphtherinum*—the diphtheria nosode—and its use as a prophylactic instead of the popular immunisation of the orthodox school. Our Homoeopathic prophylactics are far safer and are not complicated by any early or late after-effects. *Diphtherinum*, the diphtheria nosode, is an excellent preventive and has been used by other Homoeopathic physicians as well as by myself in hundreds of cases, with success.

I have given *Diphtherinum* CM in unit doses and occasionally *Diphtherinum* 30 in weekly doses for four to six weeks, and I have not heard of any failures. Of course, it may be argued that these children might not have developed it in any case—which may be true.

Which is the best potency to give for protection? I could not lay down any hard and fast rules myself; I have only been feeling my way so far. A French Homoeopathic doctor is reported to have conducted an experiment along these lines for years, and when he published his results later, he claimed that the higher potencies give longer immunity: the 1000th gave approximately two and a half years' protection, and the lower ones less, by analogy it follows that the thirtieth would protect for only a few months.

Doubt has often been expressed, whether *Diptherinum* or *any* Homoeopathic medication can truly prevent diphtheria. Records have been published by Dr. Paterson of Glasgow of the results obtained at the Mount Vernon Hospital for Children (Homoeopathic). *Diphtherinum* in the 200th potency produced definite immunity, as shown by the Schick test. All the cases done in this way gave a Schick negative result within nine weeks, and some as early as three weeks afterwards.

Dr. Mitchell reports three children who were found to be Schick positive; two doses of *Diphtherinum* in potency were given; two weeks later two of the children were Schick negative, the third became Schick negative a few weeks later, before orthodox immunisation was carried out. Dr. Mitchell adds "three cases do not prove anything except that immunity *can* be induced by Homoeopathic potencies".

Dr. Paterson was most emphatic in urging that serum should *not* be given after a Homoeopathic remedy. Very bad results had followed this method; other doctors stated that when the serum was given first, and the Homoeopathic remedy second, no evil results had followed.

Dr. Bodman said that at the Bristol Homoeopathic Hospital some thirty to forty nurses were immunised by the orthodox method. It was noticed hereafter that an enormous amount of sickness followed immediately after the immunisation. It temporarily reduced resistance to any infection, and they went down with influenza, German measles, whooping cough, and the sickness rate among the nurses was higher during the six months following diphtheria immunisation than in any period in the history of the hospital.

Personally, as I have stated already on different occasions, I have observed during the last twenty years that immunisation is followed in an appreciable percentage of cases by a general lowering of resistance, and I have seen serious and fatal cases of toxaemia coming on within a week or two after diphtheria inoculation. Dermatitis starting from the point of inoculation and spreading all over the arm and to the chest and cheek developed in three children of one family after the inoculation, and the Loeffler bacillus was found in the discharges from the skin. *Diphtherinum* M in daily doses cleared up the dermatitis in a fortnight, when previously it had gone on spreading for several months, and resisted all sorts of local treatment.

I am chary of advising diphtheria inoculations as a method of prevention of the disease. I was M.O. at a children's clinic which served a crowded area in South London within the reach of eight big schools, with a population of several hundred scholars in each. We had a daily attendance of over a hundred children for treatment. We always knew when there had been an immunisation session at any of the schools nearby, for they flocked in their dozens to us, having their swollen arms, the septic sores, and the dermatitis dressed within a few days. We used to give them—as a matter of routine—*Diphtherinum* 30 in daily doses, and got rapid healing and disappearance of the lesions. Later results in many of the children who bore the brunt of the inoculations well in the early days, were crops of multiple warts on hands, arms, and in their hundreds on the cheeks and face, peculiar dark brown, almost black, minute warts, which went on for months, but cleared up, almost overnight, at any rate in a week or two, with repeated doses of *Diphtherinum* 30.

I could fill many pages with cases of ill health of various kinds, and of fatal results, after diphtheria immunisation, during the time I was M.O. at the school clinic and at other public posts. I was not looking for serious after-effects, they came my way unsought. So from my own experience, I can only reiterate that *there is* danger from serum inoculations.

Those of us who have gone more deeply into the occult and spiritual reasons and causes of disease, know that the admixture of animal serum with human serum is not only dangerous, but wrong, and leads to long lasting effects which may take years to eradicate, and perhaps even generations—who knows? Are we not filling the blood of many thousands of people with disease products with our vaccinations and the many varieties of inoculations against all kinds of infectious diseases?

Travellers and soldiers who go abroad to the East or to the tropics, are forced to have prophylaxis against yellow fever, against cholera, against typhus, and maybe other vaccinations and inoculations. When all these different vaccinations are put into the body at more or less the same time, what confusion there must be in the serum and the body cells!

In the first world war I found, when soldiers, who had these multiple serum inoculations, later developed influenza, then it was generally a particularly virulent type which did not respond to the ordinary influenza remedies. But it did respond to *Pyrogen*, which I gave in the CM potency.

I see that Dr. Grimmer of Chicago recommends *Pyrogen* as a general antidote for multiple vaccinations. Other antidotes or prophylactics against some of the infectious diseases are: *Baptisia* against typhus and typhoid; *Arsenicum* against yellow fever; and against cholera—*Cuprum* or *Camphor* or *Veratrum Album*.

There are other prophylactics which should be made more widely known: such as against smallpox—*Variolinum*, 200 potency is best, but there are some other remedies which have proved good preventives in the past.

And now for diphtheria—it is a disease which is found commonly in temperate climes with a seasonal prevalence in autumn and late winter months, especially when there has been a deficient rainfall. It is caused by the Klebs-Loeffler bacillus and is characterised by a membranous exudate at the site of infection. It is highly infectious and may be passed from one to another by kissing or coughing and sneezing or indirectly from drinking utensils, towels, handkerchiefs, throat spatulas, and the like, that have not been properly cleansed. There are certain people who are known as carriers of the disease and they are usually immune to it themselves.

The membrane has a glistening gelatinous appearance and the tonsils are a common site for the formation. The patient complains of a sore throat, headache and general malaise. The breath has a sickening smell, and if the infection spreads, the cervical glands may become swollen and tender. Once the patient has been seen, the case can be treated along the usual lines of our Homoeopathic treatment. The patient should be confined to bed, and kept very quiet. Careful nursing is necessary so that any indication or suspicion of paralysis may be reported at once. But those Homoeopathic physicians who know their remedies have little to fear—their patients recover without the serious after-effects that so ruin the lives of many.

AILANTHUS GLANDULOSA is indicated in various zymotic disease, including diphtheria, where the patient is either semi-conscious or delirious, with a dark red, bloated or purplish face, putrid disgusting odour from the mouth. Tongue dry and brown, hacking cough. Hoarse voice.

APIS may be needed in some epidemics. Oedema of the throat and uvula, sudden stinging pains, especially on swallowing, absence of thirst, extreme aversion to heat, warm drinks and food, cold relieves greatly. The throat is bright red and puffy, and looks varnished: tongue is red, swollen and dry. Hates anything to touch the throat. *Apis* is slow in reaction and acts slowly, so should not be changed too soon. Increased flow of urine shows that it is acting favourably.

ARSENICUM—Great restlessness, fear and anguish, fear of being alone; so restless that he wants to change beds, tries to go from room to room. Great prostration, always worse at night, especially round about midnight or from 1–3 a.m.: great thirst, calling incessantly for small drinks of warm tea or hot water, inclined to vomit after drinking: all discharges putrid and foetid; great weakness and prostration. Albuminuria. Dropsy may be present, feels cold, likes heat and warm wraps, usually adapted to the later stages of the disease.

ARUM TRIPHYLLUM—indicated in nasal diphtheria. Lips, nose and angles of mouth are red and bleeding, discharge offensive and excoriating, constantly bores into the sides of the nose; tongue cracked and bleeding. Swollen submaxillary glands, irritable and restless children.

DIPHTHERINUM—Malignancy straight from the onset; in painless cases, along with epistaxis and great prostration, the membrane is thick, grey or blackish-brown. The patient is collapsed, apathetic, weak, stuporose; discharges very offensive and foetid; all the glands are swollen, vital reaction very low, sub-normal temperature. Dr. Pulford states that when the patient seems tired from the first, and the more usual remedies fail, this splendid remedy should be tried, and preferably in the CM potency.

LAC. CANINUM—Glistening, shiny red throat. *Lac. Caninum* has a tendency to go from side to side, right to left, and back again to right; the membrane is white and pearly, the coating on the tongue is milky, empty swallowing is difficult; fluids return through the nose, pains shoot into the left ear, restless dreams of snakes, skin is hypersensitive, cannot bear to be touched, is worse after a cold wind and worse after sleep; the patient is highly sensitive and imaginative, dislikes being alone; cannot bear the fingers touching one another. The main feature is alternation of sides. Both hot and cold drinks relieve inflammation of the throat.

LACHESIS—Extreme sensitiveness and intolerance of touch and pressure are the main characteristics. Intolerance of collar round the neck and neckband, or even the bed clothes; hates warm drinks, and chokes easily. The inflammation begins on the left side and travels to the right. The throat is dark and purple as well as the face; the breath is foetid; extreme prostration. A

Lachesis patient is inclined to be loquacious and suspicious, even of the doctor and any medicine that is offered. Dislikes heat and is worse after a long sleep; likes being alone. Reverse *Lac. Caninum.*

LYCOPODIUM is a nervous emotional patient who complains of the right side of the throat, pain and inflammation start on the right side extending to the left. Worse from 4 p.m. to 8 p.m. Feels the cold. Likes warm drinks, inclined to fullness and distension in the abdomen and noisy flatulence. The nose may be obstructed, the alae nasi move in a fan-like manner, must breathe through the mouth with the tongue protruded; urine is diminished, sediment is copious, consisting of fine red sand. Children waken up cross and angry, cry out during sleep.

MERCURIUS CYANATUS—Rapid onset; the main symptom is profound prostration right from the beginning; so great a weakness that standing is impossible, with coldness, cyanosis and threatening collapse. The tongue is thickly coated, breath offensive, saliva thick and ropy; the tongue may be brown, and even black. The membrane spreads rapidly over the throat, it is greenish, sometimes yellowish or grey. It apparently spreads all over the intestinal tract, for it appears even as low down as the anus. There is a tendency to destruction to the palate and the fauces. The pulse is rapid with tendency to profuse sweat. The patient is worse in the evening and at night and dislikes the heat of the bed. It is serious sign when epistaxis comes on.

PHYTOLACCA—Giddiness and nausea on sitting up, much aching of the head, back and limbs, stiffness of the muscles, and pain in the knees; the membrane is grey or white, like dirty wash-leather, usually starts

33

first on the uvula, the tongue is heavily furred, with a fiery red tip, great pain at root of tongue on putting it out; the throat is almost purple or dark red, worse with hot drinks, likes cold fluids, and the pain extends from the throat to the ears.

In the post-diphtheritic paralysis, *Gelsemium* is of greatest use when fluids regurgitate through the nose, the patient is weak, flabby, lethargic and is slow in recovering.

SCARLET FEVER

SCARLET FEVER is going through a period of decline. Like all epidemic diseases it went, in the middle of the last century, through a period of high mortality, so that scarlet fever was as much dreaded by the medical profession as by the laity. At the moment the disease incidence is low, as well as the mortality rate. In this country, cases of scarlet fever are usually referred direct to the fever hospital, so that the general practitioner has but little experience in dealing with it, but in other countries, to wit, North America, the family doctor, in the country districts at any rate, has had to deal with this epidemic disease himself. Dr. Pulford reports that in over a period of fifty-eight years of practical experience with epidemics of scarlet fever, measles, chickenpox and even diphtheria, with the help of Homoeopathic treatment he was enabled to treat these cases without any fatal results. Other physicians in North America confirm that Homoeopathy cures without any fatal results, and is not followed by any serious complications.

Scarlet fever is an acute contagious disease with fever, a characteristic inflammation of the throat and typical rash, followed by desquamation and peeling of the skin during convalescence. Incubation is from one to seven days. The onset is abrupt with vomiting, fever and sore throat which gradually increase in severity. The mucous membrane of the throat and palate become bright red with a punctate rash. The tongue is thickly furred, the enlarged inflamed papillae show through the white edges—this is the typical Strawberry

Tongue, which later changes to the Raspberry Tongue when the white furring disappears. Our early clinicians were acute observers and were fond of comparing the various characteristics of diseases to different articles of food. The skin rash appears within twenty-four hours: a bright deeply flushed face, so called "scarlet face", except for an oval white area round the bright red lips, is typical of the disease. The rash usually starts on the neck and spreads over the body and the limbs. This brightly flushed skin shows millions of minute points of the same intense red—the typical heavy punctate erythema. The rash is absent on the palms and on the soles; on the rest of the body it may persist for a week or longer. The peeling begins when the rash fades from the neck and extends down the trunk and limbs, and may continue for several weeks. Complications are glandular swelling; rhinitis; middle-ear infections; discharging ears; arthritis; nephritis, with oedema of the feet and legs, and endocarditis. The patient should be isolated until all discharges from ears, nose and eyes have disappeared.

The best known remedy in ordinary cases of scarlet fever, as well as the one most frequently indicated, is BELLADONNA. A *Belladonna* case is early recognised. The face, indeed the whole body, is burning, red and hot. The heat is so intense as to almost burn the hand which touches it. The body is scarlet, dry and smooth; there is great excitement; the eyes are red, the pupils dilated, and the carotid arteries throb violently; the mouth, the lips and throat are hot and dry, scarlet in colour; there is great thirst and restlessness; the tongue shows the typical strawberry appearance. The delirium is worse from light, noise, jarring of the bed, and motion; worse from 3 p.m. until midnight. *Belladonna* wants to be kept warm. Hahnemann already recognised the importance of *Belladonna* in scarlet fever because of its similarity to the disease, especially in cases with the smooth form of eruption.

APIS is very similar to *Belladonna*, except that the rash is thick and rough to the touch. It is thirstless and dislikes being covered; dislikes heat in any shape or form; it is averse to warm food and drink, and likes a cool room; cold relieves both the mental and physical condition. *Belladonna* reverse. The throat is oedematous, bright rosy red with stinging pain. The skin is also apt to sting and itch, causing great restlessness and weeping. The meninges may become involved; there may be rolling of the head from side to side, squinting of the eyes and then cri-encephalique (brain cry). In all oedematous cases, always consider *Apis*, and remember that *Apis* is thirstless, with a waxy skin; also in albuminuria, during desquamation, with scanty high coloured urine. So in post-scarlatinal dropsy, *Apis* may come in, even if uraemia is present.

AILTHANUS is a remedy to be considered when the eruption comes out in patches which are red and mottled. There is so much poison in the body that the vital powers are impeded and the rash is slow in coming out. The nose is stuffy, and the discharge from the nose and mouth makes the lips sore; it is also offensive. The tongue is parched and cracked. The pupils are widely dilated and sluggish; the patient is semi-conscious, dizzy, cannot sit up, and later becomes insensible with muttering delirium and stupor. *Ailanthus* belongs to the gangrenous type of malignant scarlet fever and resembles *Ammon. Carb.* and *Lachesis*. It follows well after *Rhus Tox*.

AMMON. CARB. is another remedy suitable in malignant scarlet fever. Sleepiness and somnolence are its main symptoms. The glands are swollen, the throat is dark red and sore, and the eruption is but faintly developed, face is puffy and dusky in colour. All the fluids and discharges are acrid, and the lips are excoriated. The nose is obstructed at night and the patient starts up in his sleep and lies with his mouth wide open. Great prostration, aversion to water, is usually worse at 3 a.m.; resembles a state of extreme blood poisoning. The eruption is miliary in type, and the *Ammon. Carb.* throat is dark red, while the drowsiness is more complete than in the *Belladonna* patient.

ARUM TRIPHYLLUM. You recognise this remedy by the constant working of the nostrils. The patient is busily boring and picking the nose all the time, and picking at the dry lips until they are raw and bleeding. There are red streaks from the nose to the lips. The mouth is sore and raw, the angles of the mouth are cracked and bleed, also the tongue. He refuses to take any food or drink because of the soreness of the mouth and throat. The *Arum* patient is extremely restless and very irritable. A swollen and bloated face; scanty or suppressed urine. Delirium may be present. *Arum* should not be given too low or repeated too often. Increased flow of urine shows the remedy is working well, as in *Apis*.

LACHESIS has extreme aversion to and aggravation from touch, pressure and heat, especially from touch about the throat. Cannot bear any tight pressure and hot drinks produce suffocation. Aggravation on falling asleep or after sleep, on waking up. The face, indeed the whole body becomes purple, the breath is foetid, the left side of the throat is worse and may extend over to the right. The tongue catches behind the teeth on protrusion. The child is drowsy, loquacious, delirious. Blood poisoning is present in a *Lachesis* case. It may be indicated in dropsy after scarlet fever, when there is oedema of the lower extremities, and the urine is black and scanty.

MURIATIC ACID has great muscular weakness and prostration, the jaw is hanging down; the patient slides down the bed, and later on becomes incontinent due to the paralytic weakness of anal and urethral sphincter muscles. The body intensely red like a boiled lobster, scattered, sparse rash interspersed with bluish petechia, like *Ailanthus*. Restless, cold, dislikes being covered—thin discharge trickles from the nose and burns the lips; the body turns more and more purplish; the mouth becomes studded with deep cut ulcers having a dark base. You find *Muriatic Acid* indicated in malignant scarlet fever, often complicated with diphtheria.

PHOSPHOROUS. Extreme thirst for cold drinks, the colder the better, with irritability of the stomach so that drink is vomited as soon as it gets warm. The patient is restless, apathetic and tired; generally worse from lying on the left side and from afternoon until midnight. Suitable for gangrenous types and when pneumonia is threatening. The chest feels tight, as if there was a heavy load resting on it. Suitable in cases with chest complications, bronchitis or pneumonia.

RHUS TOXICODENDRON is extremely restless, there is so much pain that movement is needed in order to ease the pains. While resting, the muscles become stiff, lame and sore, so that movement is hardly possible. Therefore the pains are worse on beginning to move. The greatest relief is from motion and heat. The throat is dark red and swollen; the tongue is red, smooth, and a triangular red tip is frequently found. The rash is coarse and dark red. *Rhus Tox.* is of use when the eruption does not come out freely, and it is dark red and coarse when it does appear. Mild delirium and dreams of hard labour may be present. *Ammon. Carb.* resembles *Rhus Tox.* but it is less restless and more somnolent. "Rely on *Rhus Tox.* when an acute disease takes on typhoid symptoms and replaces *Belladonna* when the child becomes restless and drowsy" (Farrington).

STRAMONIUM. Great violence is a predominant feature; gets excited and flies into a rage; a flushed face which looks wild and frightened; the head is hot, there is high fever, while the limbs are cold; bright light is not liked; violent hallucinations; the throat is dry, but not relieved by drinking. Suitable in convulsions alternating with rage. Restless, intense heat may lead to confusion with *Belladonna*, but *Belladonna* is not so wild, violent or so fearful.

SULPHUR is suitable in cases where all the orifices of the body are extremely red, and the discharges from the body openings are sore and burn. The lips and eyelids are red, as if they were painted, the soles of the feet are hot and burn at night, so that the covers of the bed are kicked off, or the feet are put out of bed to cool them. There may be diarrhoea at 5 a.m. in the morning, and the patient hates to be bathed or washed. There is faintness and weakness at 11 a.m. Thirsty, but not hungry. Leading remedy for a receding eruption, also when cases relapse.

TEREBINTH. Suitable in albuminuria and uraemia after scarlet fever. With dropsy, blood in urine, breathlessness and drowsiness. The patient is confused, but improves as soon as he passes water freely. Constant burning with smoky turbid urine and deposits of coffee ground sediment.

ZINCUM. Always think of *Zincum* when you find a patient persistently restless, with fidgety feet, especially at night in bed. The patient is excitable, extremely sensitive, with tendency to convulsions, a pale face and absence of heat. The head rolls from side to side, and the urine becomes suppressed. Eventually stupor and complete unconsciousness follows. Jerking during sleep with occasional screams, worse when other people talk. *Zincum* is useful in receding eruptions. The skin is livid and cold, the pulse thread-like and weak. So with fidgety feet, grinding of teeth in a pale, livid child, who screams when moved, and where the rash is slow in coming out, *Zincum* is the correct remedy.

In CUPRUM you find tendency to convulsions and spasmodic contractions, starting in fingers and toes, the flexor muscles being mainly affected; the fingers and thumbs being firmly clenched across the palms. Vomiting is often present, also stupor. Drinks gurgle down the gullet to the stomach. Frightened on waking up without recognising anybody.

MEASLES

An acute infectious disease with sharp fever and a characteristic rash which fells its victims in early childhood, and only attacks adults who have not had measles previously. The story of several attacks of this disease are unauthenticated unless supported by the evidence from a hospital, for food, drug and serum rashes are often mistaken for it by lay people. Until recently, measles was thought of as a mild affection and not worthy of the attentions of a doctor. This assumption is not always correct, for when measles hits an unsalted, non-immunised community, such as the population of the Fiji Islands was in 1875, it swept across it with extreme rapidity and killed 40,000 out of the 150,000 inhabitants.

Incubation is twenty-one days and the invasion period is two to three days. Severe catarrh of the eyes and nose with sneezing and violent dry and short coughs are the preliminary symptoms, and in this early stage it is difficult to diagnose between a simple cold and measles; both show a high infectivity. Koplik spots, like minute whitish flecks should be looked for inside the mucous membrane of the mouth. The skin rash shows itself on the third or fourth day, usually after a sleep. The temperature goes up to 103° or 104°. A smooth pink, blotchy macular rash begins behind the ears, spreads from there over the face, neck and chest; later these blotches coalesce. The appearance of a measles case is not characteristic—a puffy blotchy face, swollen eyelids, narrow palpebral fissure with injected conjunctivae, the eyelashes matted together with a thick purulent discharge. The child is miserable and unhappy; avoids the light and resents being examined. After a period of five or seven days the rash begins to fade and the temperature falls. A brownish staining of the skin remains for a few days.

In a mild attack without complications a child is well within a fortnight. Complications are unfortunately common and serious, such as, bronchitis, blepharitis, corneal ulcer, broncho-pneumonia, with emphysema of the lungs, fibrosis and cavity formation of the lung. Whooping cough is another most serious complicating factor, and the mortality rate of the combined diseases is high. Middle-ear disease and mastoid trouble, croup or laryngitis may follow, and so does diphtheria. It is difficult to control an outbreak in a school. The advice most generally given now is to isolate contacts from the ninth to the eighteenth day after infection.

A few personal notes may be suitable at this point. During several years in general practice, I went through four epidemics and amongst several hundred cases seen, I was fortunate enough with the help of Homoeopathic remedies not to lose a single case, though in the nearby neighbourhood one heard of many children who died of this disease. It was said that all my cases were extremely mild—they were mild because Homoeopathic medicines made them so.

The most usual remedies necessary in measles are: *Aconite*; *Antimonium Crudum*; *Apis*; *Arsenicum*; *Belladonna*; *Bryonia*; *Euphrasia*; *Gelsemium*; *Ipecacuanha*; *Phosphorus*; *Pulsatilla*; *Rhus toxicodendron*; *Sulphur*.

ACONITE is given as a routine measure in all kinds of fevers and high temperatures by some doctors. This habit only conduces to trouble and may delay the heal-

43

ing process. *Aconite* is indicated for a definite type of measles. A chubby, rosy, robust, well developed child is stricken down rapidly with a dry cough, some retching, intense fever, violent burning heat, great restlessness, throws himself about; much anxiety. He may have been out that day in a cold icy wind; thirst for cold water, of which he cannot get enough, glassy eyes with a red face. If you give *Aconite* to such a child the rash will come out the next day, and in two or three days that child will be well. If *Aconite* is given to an infant which has not got the red face, the restlessness and fearfulness, with great thirst, you will get no response, and you will have to change the remedy a day or two later.

ANTIMONIUM CRUDUM. An *Antimonium Crudum* measles case is very different. The child is ugly, cross and peevish; cannot bear to be touched or even looked at. The nostrils as well as the corners of the mouth are sore and cracked. He has a hot, red face, like *Aconite* it is true. There is no thirst, no anxiety, no restlessness. Instead he is delirious and drowsy. The tongue is covered with a thick slimy, milky white fur. He will retch and gag easily at any food offered to him. He objects to a hot room, or being near a hot fire.

APIS. An *Apis* case is different again. The face is puffy, swollen and red; the eyelids are swollen; the child is delirious, gradually becoming unconscious. The eyes are intensely red, face flushed; worse when the room is hot. There will be shrieking and calling out during sleep. The rash is not properly out. You might almost say there are meningeal symptoms present. The head may be drawn back and held rigidly. The child refuses hot drinks and hot applications. Give *Apis* to such a patient and the threatening meningeal symptoms and the brain cry will disappear, and the rash will come out rapidly. The temperature will go down, and within three or four days you will hardly remember that you had such a sick child to look after.

ARSENICUM has the usual symptoms of restlessness, weakness, prostration; feels chilly and wants to be well covered, with a desire for sips of hot fluid—cold drinks being refused. *Arsenicum* will clear up this case in a day or so.

BELLADONNA—See *Belladonna* under scarlet fever.

BRYONIA is perhaps the most commonly needed remedy for measles in this country. It corresponds to the tempo of measles. It comes on slowly and gradually. The symptoms take three days to develop. Symptoms of mild cold, nasal catarrh, hard dry cough; in three days the rash is fully out. The face is heavy, congested and dusky. He looks stupid and benumbed, dazed and wants to sleep all the time. He just mutters, but does not talk much unless he is disturbed, when he will rouse up and say in a disagreeable voice "Go away", and sink back to his drowsy sleep. The drowsiness and muttering delirium is worse after 9 p.m. The child wants to be left alone and wants to be kept quiet. He keeps quite still because he is worse from movement. He hates a stuffy over-heated room, he will then throw off his bedclothes and the muttering will be aggravated. On opening the windows and letting in fresh air the child will drop off to sleep quietly. The tongue is thickly coated, dry, brown and cracked, and the child has great thirst for large quantities of water at long intervals. The perspiration is free. In our damp marine climate, *Bryonia* should always be considered for all acute diseases, and it will answer well in many cases of measles, German measles and other epidemic diseases. Just one example:

A child of eleven had not felt well with a temperature for three days. The rash came out in the afternoon after the child had been drowsy all day. Temperature 104–106° at 4 p.m.; drowsy, stupid, flushed, dusky face, rouses up now and then asking for water, taking a good cupful and then lying back again to sleep. Typical dry measles cough; rhonchi all over the chest; respirations 36; pulse 148, and a high temperature as mentioned before. *Bryonia* M. in water given two-hourly. Temperature next morning 99°. The day after, thirty-six hours after the rash had come out, the temperature was normal; the rash almost gone; no pains, no headaches; chest clear; all adventitious sounds disappeared. Ravenous for food; extremely lively. Kept in bed for a couple of days. Allowed to get up on the fifth day, went out into the garden on the sixth day as it was a nice warm mild day. Seen a week later—well, and no complications followed.

EUPHRASIA is the remedy par excellence for measles with inflammation of the eyes and eyelids; catarrhal condition of the eyes with profuse burning tears; the lids of the eyes burn and itch and are swollen. Rash about the eyes with puffiness and bloating round; much sneezing and running of the nose; profuse non-irritating catarrh; the nose is streaming, more when lying down and more at night; while the dry cough is better on lying down and worse during the day; intense headache; Photophobia with a high temperature. When these symptoms are present, give *Euphrasia* 6 or 30 two-hourly in water and the temperature will be down in twenty-four to thirty-six hours; the rash will have faded in two or three days. Keep the child indoors for another two or three days in a well ventilated, airy room, protecting the eyes from too much light. Let the child go out of doors for a short time on a fine day, and there will be no chest complications, no bronchopneumonia. Inflammation of the eyes will have disappeared. There will be no falling out of the eyelashes, no disfiguring red-rimmed eyelids for months and years, with recurrent attacks of blepharitis and conjunctivitis, as is so often the case with measles treated in the orthodox fashion. This is not a fable, but fact based on experience collected over a number of years.

GELSEMIUM will be needed when measles develops during a warm, mild winter, or in a June or July epidemic. The disease comes on slowly; there is a cold with catarrh for several days; tiredness and weariness of the whole body and the limbs—the limbs are so heavy and full of weight—it is too much trouble to move them. There is a congested feeling in the head and face which looks purplish and congested. The eyes are swollen and there is profuse shedding of tears; shuddering down the back as if it were rubbed with ice. Always remember the great tiredness and weariness and disinclination to move although the cause is quite different from the disinclination for movement found in *Bryonia*, where it is due to actual pain on movement. *Gelsemium* does not move because of the weight in the limbs, neither is there any thirst nor craving for water in a *Gelsemium* case. *Gelsemium* 6 or 30 given two-hourly in water will clear up the disease in two or three days.

IPECACUANHA is indicated when there is nausea, vomiting, great weakness and prostration, with absence of thirst. The rash is slow in coming out and the gastric upset shown by the nausea and vomiting is accompanied with a flushed bright red face and clear red tongue; without any thirst. *Ipecacuanha* will stop the gastric symptoms and the dry cough. The rash will appear within a few hours as always, and the child will be well without any complications following within a couple of days.

KALI BICHROMICUM resembles *Pulsatilla*, is useful at a later stage of the disease, but the discharges from the eyes, nose and mouth are more profuse, purulent, stringy and ropy. The glands of the neck are swollen, and there is deafness due to catarrh extending to the Eustachian tubes.

PHOSPHORUS. A *Phosphorus* case is one where you find involvement of the bronchial tubes and the lungs. The respirations are rapid, the pulse and temperature are high; has great thirst for cold water; a bright red flush on the cheeks; the head is thrown back. It is a serious case and without this remedy you would expect serious trouble, but *Phosphorus* will soon alter the picture. The broncho-pneumonia will clear up in a surprisingly quick period of time, and all signs of lung involvement will disappear in twenty-four hours.

PULSATILLA has the usual measles symptoms with the rough blotchy rash, high temperature, without any thirst whatsoever. You will find a depressed, weepy and whiny child who dislikes being left alone; wants his hands held and a lot of fuss made of him; wants constant attention, so different from the *Bryonia* child; *Pulsatilla* will brighten up this child, reduce the temperature and clear up the rash within two or three days.

RHUS TOXICODENDRON. A restless child with the usual common measles symptoms. Full of aches and pains; throws himself about in bed all the time, but there is an absence of fear and anxiety. The tongue is covered with a whitish fur with a bright red tip; some thirst present.

SULPHUR is useful in a child without any particularly striking symptoms except the common measles ones— the rash; congested blotchy face; dirty tongue and perhaps an itchy skin. The child is worse in the morning about 11 a.m. *Sulphur* is often indicated in cases of measles seen late, after they have been treated by other practitioners. The weakness, debility and lack of reaction will disappear immediately *Sulphur* is given.

Kent says that "routinists do well in measles with *Pulsatilla* and *Sulphur*, occasionally requiring *Aconite* and *Euphrasia*".

MORBILLINUM is extremely useful for cases of debility, weak eyes, blepharitis, conjunctivitis, etc., left after severe measles. Treated in fever hospitals, children who simply will not put on weight, are anaemic, weary, and often with some bronchitis, *morbillinium* will help to remove all these symptoms, prevent lung complications and help them to assimilate their food well and to put on weight rapidly.

A final word for those who may not have dealt with the case from the start. In suppressed eruption where the brain is affected, remember *Apis*, *Zinc*, *Stramonium* and *Cuprum*, where there are cramps, convulsions, spasms of the fingers and toes, and when the patient starts in his sleep. Also think of *Hellebore* when the child lies in a state of deep unconsciousness from which he can hardly be roused.

INFLUENZA

INFLUENZA is a highly infectious epidemic disease of protean character which affects the upper respiratory tract. It occurs periodically in minor waves of thirteen to fifteen weeks. If such a wavelet coincides with cold inclement weather, the outbreak may affect a number of susceptible persons. In between these periodic outbreaks it seems to disappear entirely. Then there are the outbreaks of a more virulent type which occur in the first three months of every two years when the mortality rate goes up considerably. For the last 100 years approximately there have been pandemics, i.e. epidemics which spread across whole continents with lightning rapidity at intervals of thirty years. Some may still recall the pandemic of 1889 and '90, and many will have vivid recollections of the 1918–20 epidemic which was world wide and carried off thousands of war-weary victims. We are now in the midst of another outbreak which has already shown a high death rate. Under orthodox treatment the mortality rate is from 25–30 per cent, especially if the lungs become affected, and even the vaunted sulphonamides and penicillin do not lower it much.

It strikes its victims down like lightning, and unlike the virus diseases, one attack predisposes another. The incubation period is one to three days at the most, and it is highly infectious in the early catarrhal stage. The principal symptoms are headache, sore throat and severe pain in limbs and back with a high temperature. It is the fashion to call every slight feverish chill influenza; but if after the temperature has come down, the depression, exhaustion and weariness is such that it is too much effort to do anything, that life is really not worth living, you know you have had influenza; after a mere feverish chill you will feel as well on getting up as you did before the attack. Unfortunately many people take no notice of the danger signals of weakness and prostration, and insist on getting up, even returning to work before they are fit, thus laying themselves open to broncho-pneumonia and sudden death.

During the 1918–20 epidemic the mortality rate was 30 per cent and 25,000 people died in America alone under orthodox treatment, while the Homoeopathically treated members of the community showed a death rate of under 1 per cent. It is a pity that these figures which show such staggering differences are never referred to or made known to the general public. A system of treatment which cures people so rapidly and thoroughly is well worth investigation in my opinion. The trouble is firstly ignorance of the true facts of the case, secondly disbelief in their truth, and thirdly, as far as the doctors are concerned, the great difficulty is differentiating between the various remedies needed to cure a sick person rapidly and efficiently. As always, it is necessary to study each case clinically at the bedside and carefully collect the symptoms presented by the individual. This takes time; it is so much easier to walk into a room, diagnose the case, and write out the prescription of the prevalent fashionable drug. The Homoeopathic doctor has to know his Materia Medica with all its drugs exceedingly well before he can match up with the correct remedy the symptoms shown by the sick person. He has to take so many factors into consideration. There are quite thirty to forty remedies for influenza, and to find the right one which will cut short the feverish attack and permit the patient to feel well without complications following within a few days, is extraordinarily difficult. One should be able to reduce the temperature and remove the pains and all the acute symptoms within twenty-four to forty-eight hours at the most. After that, even though the temperature remains normal, it is essential that the patient remains in bed for five days at the least, and if at all possible, for a week. During the feverish period the patient should be allowed nothing but raw fruit and fruit juices, and *not* synthetic bottled juices. Fresh oranges, lemon juice, apple drinks, grapefruit drinks at frequent intervals will cleanse the system and prevent any undue strain being thrown on the gastric organs. No meat juices, no milk, are permissible. After the temperature is down, the diet may be increased and may include vegetable broth, Yeastrel drinks, wholemeal toast; gradually other foods may be added, such as milk dishes, fish, chicken, salads, as the patient desires. Under such a regime you will find there is no constipation. No laxatives should ever be given during a feverish attack or any infectious disease. With a fruit diet such as mentioned, nature will reassert herself in a few days and the rhythmic contractions of the gastro-intestinal tract will return to normal. It may take three, four or five days, but this is nothing to be alarmed about, because during a high temperature the normal metabolism is so deranged that there are very few waste products left. Nature burns up many of the poisons and impurities in the system; it is a kind of bonfire taking place in the body which will consume and reduce to the simple chemical elements the various fats and proteins taken in by and stored in the body.

As already mentioned, there is a choice of remedies for the Homoeopathic doctor to select from. In cold wet spells the remedies needed would be *Bryonia, Dulcamara, Allium Cepa, Pulsatilla*; in a mild warm spell, it would be *Eupatorium, Gelsemium, Pyrogen*; *Arseni-*

cum is a very common remedial drug in catarrhal influenza. In cold dry windy weather, *Aconite, Causticum, Hepar Sulphuris* and *Nux Vomica* have to be considered. The nosode *Influenzinum* works very well given night and morning in conjunction with one of the indicated acute remedies mentioned.

It is not a wise plan to give *Aconite* in every case at the beginning of a feverish chill, as the lay people are so fond of doing. *Aconite* should only be given, if a chill develops after exposure to a cold dry wind, when the patient is smitten within a few hours of exposure, with a hot burning face, and other *Aconite* symptoms —extreme restlessness, agonised tossing about, great fear—especially fear of dying, and faint feeling on getting up or sitting up. If a combination of these symptoms is present, *Aconite* will answer well; if not, it is a mere waste of time.

During influenza, ARSENICUM is really indicated in this country much more than *Aconite*—if given diluted in water every two hours at first and later four-hourly, it would cut short many an attack, and bring the temperature down in twelve hours or so. In *Arsenicum* there is restlessness, prostration, weakness, pains, headaches and backache, great thirst for frequent sips of warm drinks and general aggravation after midnight.

ALLIUM CEPA. After exposure to cold damp wind, with bland watery discharge from the eyes, and excoriating discharge from the nose. Throat and larynx are raw extending into the chest; tickling cough and tearing pain in larynx with cough—usually left-sided nasal catarrh.

BAPTISIA. Comes on rapidly, prostration, stupidity, mottled face, bleeding and putrid mouth; the patient looks as if he were drunk; confused, delirious, disassociated, feels that there are two of him; his limbs are scattered, restless, tosses and turns.

BRYONIA is a common remedy for influenza. You expect to see a sleepy, heavy, lethargic patient with a flushed contused face, who dislikes being disturbed; a thickly coated tongue, is thirsty for large drinks of cold water at rare intervals. Has backache, headache, eyeache, aching limbs, is worse from movement, so he lies still and does not move. There is profuse perspiration; he feels under the weather for several days before the disease fully develops. The pace of the complaint is slow.

EUPATORIUM PERFOLIATUM is a remedy for warm mild weather. The most outstanding symptom is the extreme aching right deep in the bones, the back and the legs—feeling as if the bones would break; the patient is restless; there is no comfortable place in bed; it feels hard. Coated tongue. There is great heat but no perspiration. *Bryonia* and *Eupatorium* can be easily mistaken one for the other, but if you remember that *Bryonia* lies quietly and does not like to be disturbed, and *Eupatorium* is restless, you are less likely to confuse the two.

GELSEMIUM is also a remedy in a warm mild winter, or in the summer. It is usually associated with a nervous shock, fear or fright or emotional upset. Great exhaustion, weariness, prostration, so tired he cannot exert himself to move or turn round; wants to be left alone. Face suffused and congested. Thirstless.

HEPAR SULPHURIS. In cold dry windy weather, in north and north-east winds. He feels cold in the back of the neck on moving. There is stitching pain in the throat; he is sensitive to any kind of pain; irritable, nasty tempered to those near him. Needs to cover back of neck with woollen shawl even in bed. Profuse perspiration. Difficult patient mentally, always complaining about everybody that comes near.

NUX VOMICA is needed after exposure to a cold east or north-east wind. The patient feels cold, shivers, shivers from motion, moving bedclothes will bring on a shivering attack. Patient is disagreeable, bad tempered, snappy, wants to be left severely alone. Aching in all limbs, severe headache, eyeache, worse moving eyes or turning to the light, prefers the dark. Nausea and thickly coated tongue.

PULSATILLA. Attack comes on after getting wet and getting wet feet. Shivers up and down the back, with high temperature—feeling of cold water pouring down the back. There is much catarrh and congestion in back of nose and throat, and the patient feels worse in a warm, stuffy room; prefers fresh air; is worse in the evenings; high temperature with dry mouth and no thirst.

PYROGEN is again similar to *Eupatorium*. It has the deep aching in the bones—excessive restlessness, he has to move, although it hurts; the bed is uncomfortable and hard. There is profuse perspiration, the bed is soaked rapidly, the patient is delirious, he is always looking round for parts of his body, that is, he has too many legs, etc., in his delirium. There is usually a strong septic element as the exciting cause of the disease. There is dissimilarity (which is typical of this medicine) in the pulse/temperature ratio—a high temperature of 103° and a pulse of 80, or a temperature of 99–100° and a pulse of 140–150.

RHUS TOXICODENDRON after exposure to wet. Aching in all limbs; worse on beginning to move, very restless, has to go on moving, if he keeps still the pain and aching gets worse; cannot find a restful place in bed. Tongue coated, with a red triangle at front of tongue.

One often forgets *Causticum* which is indicated in cold dry easterly winds. Neuralgic pains, face-ache; dry hollow cough, producing escape of urine. A sip of cold water relieves cough. Limbs feel as if they have been beaten. Chilliness during temperature followed by perspiration without an intermediate hot stage.

Weakness, prostration and excessive exhaustion after influenza, with easy perspiration on movement, warm wet hands, disinclined to exert oneself, is normally covered by KALI PHOS. 6 three times a day for several days, or four doses of *Kali Phos.* 200, strictly *only* four doses of the 200th potency, given night and morning. In a few cases it has been noted that two doses only are necessary. Homoeopathic medicines should never be continued after improvement is established. *Kali Phos.* acts like champagne and puts new life into the patient and dispenses with seaside convalescence.

In some cases influenza acts as a severe nerve poison. It may leave a great depression, almost suicidal in character; even in people who are well balanced as a rule. In such a contingency *Cypripedium* 6 three times a day will remove this unpleasant and serious trouble.

Complications do not usually occur with Homoeopathic treatment but are not unknown after allopathic medicines. One often sees people who trace back many of their chronic disabilities to an attack of influenza. In these cases remember INFLUENZINUM 30 or 200, given at weekly intervals until improvement sets in. Deafness coming on slowly, insidiously and progressively after an attack of influenza may often be alleviated and improved by *Influenzinum* 30 or 200.

Recurrent attacks of influenza, when a patients falls a victim, whenever he or she comes within the orbit of the disease will be cured by TUBERCULINUM 30, given once every ten days for six doses. These doses may have to be repeated in the autumn months, every ten to fourteen days during October, November and December.

MUMPS

Mumps is a benign, highly contagious feverish disease associated with a swelling of the parotid gland. It is due to a virus, and attacks mainly children about five years of age and young adolescents. Whenever it breaks out, it runs like wild fire through communities of young people, schools, barracks, scout camps and offices. The incubation period is from twenty-one to thirty days, and isolation and quarantine should be practised for twenty-one days. The preliminary symptoms are a slight nasal catarrh with a rise of temperature to 102° or 103°, tenderness of the area around the ears, followed by a unilateral swelling of the parotid. The gland on the other side usually enlarges a day or two later. There is pain during mastication and even on opening the mouth. The contour of the face is altered completely as the hollows of the neck near the lobe of the ears and the lower jaw are filled up by the swelling of the glands. This gives the patient a somewhat ludicrous appearance which will rouse the risibility of his friends.

Mumps produces more errors of diagnosis than almost any other epidemic disease. Lay people, teachers, nurses, and parents find it difficult to distinguish between mumps and swellings of the glands of the neck, but even general practitioners frequently err in this respect by wrongly diagnosing swollen cervical glands associated with inflamed tonsils, as mumps, and most serious mistakes can be made by diagnosing the bull-neck of toxic diphtheria as mumps. It should be essential for doctors in every case of childish complaints to look carefully into the throat for signs of diphtheric infections. It should be remembered that swollen glands are always movable and extend respectively either above or below the border of the lower jaw, while a swollen parotid anatomically lies in front, below and behind the lobe of the ear, surrounded by a fixing capsule, so that a swollen parotid is hard, tense, immovable and circumscribed.

Mumps is often complicated by orchitis, inflammation of the testicles, in 25–40 per cent of the cases, while ovarian infection and mastitis is only found in 5–8 per cent. Encephalitis, involvement of the cerebral spinal nervous system, is occasionally found. This is said to be a frequent serious complication in China, and the Far East.

The orthodox treatment of mumps is largely expectant—rest, warmth, isolation, and sedatives if pain is severe. In the early days of my practice I followed this regime. As a house surgeon in one of the Homoeopathic hospitals I met some cases of mumps in the isolation ward. The medicinal treatment was *Belladonna*, alternating with one of the *Mercurial* preparations. Two of the girls out of three developed ovarian trouble, which made life a misery for them for many years, and I know it made one of them an invalid for several days every month for the next fifteeen years. The clinical results in these instances were not any better with Homoeopathy than with ordinary expectant treatment of the orthodox school. Homœopathy I considered a failure in mumps. Years later I came across Dr. Burnett's interesting booklets on Homoeopathic treatments of many different diseases. In more than one he stated that *Pilocarpine*, in one of the lower potencies, was a specific for parotid disease, especially mumps. During my days of apprenticeship in Homoeopathy I had heard derogatory remarks made about Burnett's writings and I had never put myself out to investigate the truth of these statements, which I have regretted very deeply ever since, for there are many treasures locked up in those little books which are well worth following up. Burnett was so positive about the benefit of *Pilocarpine* in mumps that I felt it was worth while to experiment with it in the next case I might see. *Pilocarpine* reminded me of one of the lectures on Materia Medica of a very ancient doctor in Edinburgh who was very proud of the fact that he had personally experimented with *Jaborandi*, the South American plant which is the alkaline spirit of PILOCARPINE. His vivid description of the excessive flow of saliva while he went to sleep after taking large doses of *Jaborandi* was most amusing, and became a byword amongst fresh generations of students and always produced roars of laughter when this point in the lectures was reached. The effects produced on this doctor proved to me that *Pilocarpine* certainly had a definitely violent action on the salivary glands, and following our Homoeopathic Law of Similars—producing a disturbance of the parotid in a healthy prover, it should cure inflammation of the same glands in one who was sick. A boy arrived shortly afterwards at the children's clinic, sent there by the sister of the surgical dispensary, with a provisional diagnosis of mumps. He had a temperature of 102.8°, bi-lateral swellings of the parotid gland, which was tender to touch, and with pain on opening the mouth. *Pilocarpine* 6 night and morning was prescribed, and the mother was told to bring him back to the dispensary in three days. When she turned up she remarked that the boy had mumps. Without thinking I retorted sharply "Who said so? There is no swelling at all." I was somewhat taken aback when she triumphantly answered "You did yourself on Monday afternoon." Then I remembered the little boy and to my surprise I had to admit that all signs of mumps, pain, temperature and swelling had disappeared completely in three days—a thing I had never known to happen before. After that, *Pilocarpine* 6 became the routine treatment in mumps of which we experienced quite an extensive epidemic during that year, and *Pilocarpine* 6 did not disappoint me, except in one case where the indications for *Mercurius* were so striking—prostration, heavy sweats, offensive breath, thickly coated tongue, that one could not fail to notice the similarity between the disease and the remedy, which cured the child in six days. So unless there are strong symptoms for another remedy in the nondescript common cases of mumps, *Pilocarpine* is the best and most similar remedy, and in the course of years I have had no occasion to change my opinion. It cures mumps rapidly and efficiently, and prevents it, if taken once a day for ten to twelve days by those who have been in contact with this disease.

Parotidinum 30, the nosode of mumps, helps in those cases where ill health can be traced back to a severe attack of mumps. Some observant people will tell you— "I have never been well since mumps—I have had ovarian trouble or nervous trouble, or inflammation of the testicles since an attack of mumps many years ago". This nosode in potency 30 or 200 given at intervals of ten to fourteen days will do a great deal to put these people on the road to recovery.

Some cases of mumps are followed by extreme nervous depression, and almost suicidal melancholia for three to six months after an attack. Whether this is due entirely to the congestion of the nerves caused by the virus, or whether it is due to the large doses of sedatives which are frequently prescribed by the attending practitioners, I would not care to say. Anyhow I have found *Parotidinum* extremely useful in clearing up this distressing melancholic depression.

One lady was converted to Homoeopathy by the

successful action of *Parotid* 30 in mumps. In the beginning of her married life, her husband, being a keen Homoeopath, tried hard to convert her to it. She showed the usual condescending, slightly superior attitude of the majority of the people towards Homoeopathy until her child, and she herself, developed mumps. *Parotid* 30 night and morning from the word go, and what appeared to be a severe attack of the disease, cleared up in under five days!

The mother was particularly impressed with the fact that she suffered no more pain after the first dose of the nosode, and was able to eat solid food, even crisp apples, without the slightest discomfort. She is now an enthusiastic follower of our art. Homoeopathy must be experienced on oneself in order to be fully appreciated in its full beauty.

WHOOPING COUGH (or Pertussis)

AN acute epidemic infectious disease affecting the air passages with spasms of a characteristic type of cough combined with vomiting. Etiology, Bordet-Gengou bacillus closely related to the Pfeiffer's bacillus is held to be the cause of the infection. Although it resembles a virus infection, the incubation period is long, there are no carriers, the immunity lasts for life after an attack.

Incubation period uncertain—varies from one to two weeks. Isolation four weeks at least after the first whoop is noticed, a period of six weeks is said to be safer. Contagion is due to droplet infection of saliva ejected during fits of coughing.

Symptoms—the first, or catarrhal stage lasts two weeks and shows itself as a nasal catarrh with cough worse at night and slight fever. The cough increases in intensity until it becomes more and more spasmodic in character. The second stage is the stage of paroxysms. The child is frightened, tries to sit up and hold on to the side of the cot for support or cling to his mother or nurse. There is a preliminary inhalation which resembles a long whistle followed by short suffocating spasms of cough, during which the colour of the face becomes more livid and suffused, finishing off with the well known whoop. Suddenly it almost appears as if the child would suffocate with each spasm. After several such spasms the child manages to bring up some thick slimy muco-pus and the paroxysm often ends in vomiting. The child is totally exhausted after each spasm, but soon recovers, and is happy and cheerful in between the attacks. There may be as many as forty to fifty attacks a day, and owing to the exhaustion and the constant vomiting, the metabolism may be severely interfered with. Sublingual ulcer is commonly found due to the friction of the tongue against the teeth during a paroxysm. Marasmus is a common sequel to whooping cough. Touching the base of the tongue with a spatula usually brings on a paroxysm, hence it may be used as a means of differential diagnosis. After four to five weeks the spasms gradually become less and less, the cough is more productive and the phlegm looser. This third stage may last another two to three weeks, though in not a few cases these spasms of coughing may go on for a few months, and with each fresh cold, for the next twelve months, whenever a cough recurs, the spasms of typical whoops may appear again as well, especially if the child is thwarted or annoyed.

Complications are convulsions in infants, lung abscess, empyema, late sequela, may be tuberculosis of the lung or bronchiectasis. Measles is easily contracted during pertussis (whooping cough) and the combination of these two diseases is generally unfavourable. Children under a year generally succumb to these diseases. Convulsions are a serious sign. Broncho-pneumonia is generally fatal and so is enteritis.

Parents are frequently most careless and complacent about whooping cough. One has often seen young children suffering from this complaint in playgrounds, city parks, and in public vehicles, spluttering, choking, coughing and whooping, spreading their infection to all around. Few realise how serious the disease can be and that the death rate of whooping cough was twice as high as that of measles, or even diphtheria, in the L.C.C. hospitals during the decade before the second world war.

Now treatment—during the early years of my professional life I had no opportunity to treat whooping cough. Parents accepted as a fact that whooping cough lasted at least six weeks, or until well on in May, and as it could not be cured it just had to be endured. A doctor was rarely called in. One day I procured a copy of Dr. Clarke's monograph on *Pertussin*, the nosode of whooping cough (the potentised serum of this disease). My eyes were opened to the possibilities of cutting short an epidemic of this dread disease. At that time there was a small outbreak in the neighbourhood of the clinic, so with the help of the visitors and nurses, we coaxed the mothers to bring the little sufferers to the clinic for treatment before the commencement of the session to avoid infecting others. The results with *Pertussin* in potency were so striking that I soon used it in all the clinics and nurseries I attended, both as a prophylactic and as the curative remedy after the disease had started. During the four years before the second world war, 250 cases were treated with the following results. One baby five months old died. Two mothers, having four children between them, did not carry on with the treatment after twenty-four hours, preferring their children to be sent to a fever hospital. These four youngsters were away from their homes for well over four months and came back a mere shadow of their former selves, requiring several months' convalescence at the seaside. While the children in the same street who had been dosed with the small pilules of *Pertussin* were fully recovered after only a fortnight. It created quite a stir in that neighbourhood at the time, I believe. The severity of the attacks was mitigated at once. They diminished in frequency as well. Vomiting became less violent, and the duration was considerably shortened. It depended largely on the stage of the disease at which the treatment commenced. It was aborted under a week if seen within the first day or two. If seen at its height, it would take another ten to fourteen days at the most, with greatly diminished severity. All the children escaped the usual complications. No bronchopneumonia followed, and we saw no wasting and no marasmus. It was indeed surprising how well they looked at the end of the attack—they were often better after the whooping cough than they had been before. Let me quote a typical case.

A five-year-old child after a week of catarrhal difficulties began to whoop two days before Christmas. Being a well-to-do family, the doctor was contacted at once, and he prescribed some suitable sedative. The child got steadily worse, having between thirty to forty vomiting attacks a day, thus disturbing the mother's rest considerably at night. The 2nd of January, ten days later, *Pertussin* 30 three times a day was ordered. A week later the report was that the attacks were less severe, the vomiting only slight, about once daily. The mother's sleep was hardly disturbed, she had to get up only once during the night instead of every half-hour. The local practitioner visited at the end of the month for a check-up and was so delighted with the progress of the child that he congratulated the mother on her good nursing! He had never seen a child with whooping cough recover so quickly, and without showing any signs of wasting or anaemia; indeed the weight was better at the end of the attack than before.

PROPHYLAXIS. *Pertussin* 30 acts well as a protective against whooping cough. 364 cases were given daily doses of *Pertussin* for two weeks after contact. Many of these cases were seen in the day nurseries under my care —not one of these children developed the disease. As two of the nurseries took in children from two weeks old, it was most essential that they should not be exposed to the infection, and it was gratifying to find that

Pertussin was a means of preventing the spread of the disease. To quote an early experience—When I was not sure yet of the power of *Pertussin* in preventing the disease, a girl of five years old attended a private school —of the twenty-one children in her class, eighteen were infected with a severe type of whooping cough. Only three escaped—two had had whooping cough a year before, and the third was my little friend. How anxious I was whether my little doses would work, and great was the triumph when we were successful. The school doctor, whose own two children were attacked with a particularly severe variety of whooping cough after doses of prophylactic serum administered by himself, was wrath with the little girl's mother, because he would have it that the little one must have had whooping cough the year before without the mother knowing! He accused her of not being exactly truthful as it was impossible to prevent whooping cough.

In another private school, a child came back after the holidays with a fully developed whooping cough, in spite of carrying a doctor's certificate as being free from any infectious disease. All the twelve children in her class were infected. The headmistress, on my advice, gave *Pertussin* 30 four-hourly, and the children had the mildest attack of whooping cough she had ever seen. They enjoyed being ill, playing all the time in the orchard and in the big old barn instead of having lessons. Ten years previously, she told me, whooping cough was inadvertently taken to her school. All the children had it. Weeks of great anxiety and hard work followed. Several night and day nurses had to be called in—it was a nightmare time for her. She was grateful to Homoeopathy, and to the nosode *Pertussin* for turning so serious a disease into a mild one.

The Homoeopathic doctor is always accused by his orthodox friends of only presenting single cases of cure, in support of his claim that Homoeopathic medicines prescribed according to the Law of Similars, are superior to the remedies prescribed according to the latest orthodox fashion, such as the various *sulphona-mides*, the ever lengthening list of anti-biotic remedies, the different *penicillins*, etc., but here is a case in point where a fairly substantial number of children were seen and treated successfully with the potentised nosode of whooping cough with a practically 100 per cent success. Could the orthodox physician attending similar cases of this disease show an equally successful result of his labours with the recognised multiplicity of remedies one sees in the latest text books?

RUBELLA (German Measles)

AN acute epidemic infectious disease, milder in type than measles and in some instances difficult to distinguish. It is characterised by fever, rash and a general swelling of the lymph glands, especially of the sub-occipital and posterior cervical region (back of the neck).

The cause is a filterable virus. The incubation period is fourteen to twenty-three days. It occurs mainly in young adults and older children. Incidence is particularly great wherever there is a collection of young men and women thrown together for hours, especially in offices and barracks. The incidence rate of Rubella rose considerably during the war years 1914–1918 and again during the 1939–1945 war. Because of its infectious character all cases should be isolated until the fading of the rash.

Invasion is benign, there are no premonitary symptoms—perhaps a little headache, some stiffness of the muscles of the neck, which may be attributed to a chill. There may be a little running of the nose, and some dryness of the throat. The rash shows first on the face and neck, then it attacks the trunk and the limbs. The region round the mouth is also attacked, and consists of pink, fine eruptions in between the coarse pointed scarlet fever rash and the blotches of measles. The enlarged glands may show before the rash or accompany it; they are usually, as already mentioned, in the sub-occipital glands below the hairline, the glands in the posterior triangle of the neck, and the mastoid glands. The glands in the axilla and the inguinal region are not frequently involved. A pink eye may be present, which is similar but not so intensely inflamed as the conjunctivitis in measles, and there is no discharge, no weeping, no lachrymation. Complications are rare, there may be slight bronchitis, a mild otitis media with deafness may follow.

In the last few years it has been noticed that rubella causes trouble when it occurs during pregnancy, especially if the disease develops during the first eight to twelve weeks after conception. During the last few years reports have come in from the Antipodes, Australia and New Zealand, and also here in Britain, that congenital defects in the embryo follow after infection in the mother especially such diseases as congenital cataracts, deafness, deaf mutism and congenital heart disease develop in infants where the mother had rubella during pregnancy. So it would appear wise to warn an expectant mother to avoid any contact with rubella cases in the early months of pregnancy.

Treatment: Prophylactic—PULSATILLA 6 night and morning for ten to fourteen days after contact with other cases.

When the disease develops, treat symptomatically:

ACONITE 6 for high temperature and thirst.

COFFEA 6 two to three-hourly will help if there is sleeplessness, wakefulness and sensitivity to sounds.

PULSATILLA 6 or 30 four-hourly for temperature and fever without thirst, with depression and fretfulness.

CHICKENPOX

CHICKENPOX is a mild infectious disease with a characteristic skin eruption; closely related to shingles or herpes zoster, so if one member of a family develops chickenpox, another, usually an adult, may show signs of shingles about the same time. The incubation period is two to three weeks, and isolation should be until all the scabs have fallen off.

Severe chickenpox has often been mistaken for smallpox and vice versa—an error of judgement not devoid of serious consequences. Therefore as chickenpox cases are not always brought to a doctor for diagnosis in the early stages, it behoves both doctor and lay people in my opinion to note the difference between a comparatively mild complaint without any complications and any fatal results, as chickenpox, to one which is more serious, and which is often disastrous to the sufferer, as smallpox.

(1) The eruption shows itself on the trunk and most thickly on the chest and back; it spreads to the face and arms. It shows more on the body than on the face, and more thickly on the shoulders and upper arms than on the wrists and hands; more on the thighs than on the legs, feet and soles. It is centripetal rather than centrifugal. Smallpox on the other hand is centrifugal in distribution—more on face and scalp than on the body; more on the wrists, palms and forearms than on the upper arms; more on the feet and legs than on the thighs. The hollow parts such as behind the knees and in front of the elbows are avoided and the rash more visible on prominences.

(2) In chickenpox, fresh crops of spots appear every two days preceded by or simultaneous with a rise of temperature, so you find spots in various stages of development present at the same time. Clear blisters or vesicles like drops of water lie superficially on the skin, varying in size—some are large, the size of half a pea, others are small as a pin-point; dried up crusts and scabs show at the same time. This is totally different from smallpox, where the pocks are all at the same stage of development—all vesicles, or all crusts, according to the duration.

(3) In chickenpox the spots are soft to the touch, while in smallpox the lesions are deep-set, hard and gritty to feel and are umbilicated and divided by sepsis. So in a disease where fresh crops appear every two days, you find blisters, crusts and scabs at the same time, and these are more numerous on the trunk, the rash is itchy and irritating—chickenpox is the diagnosis.

Smallpox may unfortunately be modified if the patient has been vaccinated once or twice in his lifetime, and though it may be mild in his case, he may pass it on, and be the beginning of a severe outbreak of smallpox.

ANTIMONIUM TARTARICUM is almost a specific for chickenpox. The patient is drowsy, perspires freely, there is nausea, the eruption is slow in coming out, and *Antimonium Tart.* will accelerate it. Sometimes complications with bronchitis. This remedy will rapidly break up the lung trouble.

MERCURIUS may be required if the vesicles suppurate and discharge purulent matter, with great weakness, easy sweating, and the patient feels worse at night.

RHUS TOXICODENDRON has intense itching, restlessness, and in many cases will make the eruption disappear rapidly.

SULPHUR may be needed where the patient is weak and prostrated, has no appetite, and is slow to recover.

POLIOMYELITIS

POLIOMYELITIS is another serious disease which confronts the medical profession. The Homoeopathic doctors can show successful cures founded on their Law of Similars proved on healthy individuals. Sickness means increased sensitivity of the patient to drugs and the other recognised modern means of treatment such as the serums and vaccines, hence their useless effects and sometimes fatal results. When faced with a different problem some are inclined to say there is no solution but might there not be a cleverer fellow round the corner, who has a wider vision and a little more knowledge? These fellows who have added the knowledge obtained by drug experimentations on healthy persons to the training received at the universities, colleges and hospitals, find that this expanded view of drug treatment helps them to conquer disease in a way which makes the task of healing a great joy.

Homoeopathic treatment by the application of its science of practical facts has enabled its devotees to cure thousands of cases of paralysis and nervous diseases which have troubled humanity during the last hundred years, and we have always been willing and anxious to pass on our knowledge to that great majority of our medical brethren who have not heard of it.

Infantile paralysis is one of the modern varieties of a disease which has come to the forefront during the last fifty to sixty years; gradually it has become more frequent and more virulent. It has extended its battle front for at first it attacked mainly infants and young children under two years of age; in Europe we had sporadic cases cropping up here and there, who came under the care of the orthopaedic surgeon, when paralysis set in, usually too late for the physician to deal with it. As the decades of this century have flown by, men in the twenties and thirties and older have been attacked by this insidious disease, which strikes and fells men and women overnight. The best known example of this disease is the late President Roosevelt who was attacked in his thirties, and in spite of his great disabilities, strove and worked on, nothing daunted, and became the great war leader of the United States. A shining example of victory of mind over matter.

The Homoeopathic medico working on the facts observed on healthy people taking certain drugs, found that the remedy *Lathyrus Sativus*, presented a picture in its symptomatology, strikingly alike, both pathologically and clinically to infantile paralysis, hence its use as a preventive in this disease. And it has had one hundred per cent success during the last thirty years in many epidemics, as Dr. Grimmer of Chicago, for one, states. His recommendation is: to give a dose of *Lathyrus Sativus* 30th or 200th potency once every three weeks during an epidemic, and he states there *will be no* case of paralysis among those so immunised. Does this sound too good to be true? Try it my friends and see.

The papers in Britain are full of news of the increase in the number of infantile paralysis cases; in Birmingham, the Isle of Wight, Lincoln. The number attacked in 1950 is much larger, almost twice as many as in the year 1949 and the death rate is also going up at the same time. It has started earlier in the year and it is feared that its peak has not yet been reached, for the maximum danger period is during the harvest months, September and October. Dr. Newsholme, Birmingham's

75

Medical Officer of Health, said, "Medical opinion suggests that there is a possibility of some association between poliomyelitis and certain inoculations. The exact nature of such association is not yet known. During epidemics of poliomyelitis the virus is not fully developed and many people are carriers without developing any recognisable signs or symptoms of the disease. In a number of such persons inoculations are usually followed within thirty days by some degree of paralysis." On the advice of the Ministry of Health, schemes for immunisation against diphtheria have been temporarily suspended in order to avoid such cases.

Well, *Lathyrus Sativus* is the answer to the prevention of the spread of this dread disease. This remedy has, to quote Dr. Grimmer again, "the same affinity to the same centres in the spinal cord and brain as the virus of poliomyelitis and is the most perfect antidote both for prevention and cure".

Dr. Taylor Smith of Johannesburg has recently gone through an epidemic and sent a report of his experiences to London and I shall quote largely from his report—In the early stages of the disease he claims that *Belladonna, Gelsemium, Physostigma* and *Lathyrus* are the best remedies for treatment. The onset is insidious and instantaneous. The variations are from a mild coryza (cold) to a rapid paralysis; usually there is some depression, malaise, diarrhoea, sore throat, headache, vomiting, pain and tenderness in the limbs. The umbilicus is displaced. In the early stages there is a great resemblance to influenza. In the past many cases may have been diagnosed as influenza when they were really cases of poliomyelitis.

Of course we do not depend on diagnosis alone for our treatment and so those remedies which resemble the clinical condition at that moment should be employed; and it might well be that *Gelsemium* or even

76

Eupatorium might cover the disease picture and prove to be the correct remedy to break up the disease in its early stages.

In the pre-paralytic stages one may find a curious kind of febrile invasion during which there may be an interval of three or four days, when the temperature drops to normal, then a second bout of fever returns, the temperature goes up, and you get thus the double hump or dromedary chart. General hypersensitiveness to touch is found frequently with irritability, apprehensiveness and excessive dread of being handled. There is a fine tremor of the affected muscles (*Gels.*), and the spine is so tender that the child will not flex it, a sign which makes it difficult to differentiate from the rigidity of the neck in meningitis. A typical classical sign is the "tripod" position that is the back is held rigid and straight, the trunk leans backwards on the arms, which are firmly braced to support the body. He is unable to "kiss his knees" in this position, and this is a valuable diagnostic test.

In the majority of cases paralysis comes on suddenly on the first or second day. This flaccid type of paralysis shows itself in loss of voluntary movement in the affected muscles due to oedema pressing on the sound cells, so it appears much more extensive at first than later, when recovery of these sound cells takes place after the oedema subsides, usually in a week or so. In a simple spinal case, death is uncommon, but bulbar paralysis—which is found in 20 per cent of the cases in an epidemic and is highly fatal, is due to paralysis of the respiratory muscles, which is commonly preceded by involvement of the palatal and pharyngeal muscles. So you get regurgitation of liquids through the nose. Coughing and spluttering is an early sign; in this it resembles diphtheria.

Therefore a respirator or artificial lung is now employed in these cases of respiratory difficulties in order to help the patients over this difficult stage. Once the breathing becomes normal again, this danger is over; for no residual palsy remains in this kind of case.

Now to go back to Dr. Taylor Smith's record. He used *Lathyrus Sativus* as a prophylactic in a group of eighty-two healthy people. Each was given one dose of *Lathyrus Sativus* 30, which was repeated in sixteen days; the group included forty-two white children, twenty-one coloured children, and nineteen white adults. The ages in the group varied from six months to twenty years; moreover they all lived in close proximity to a suspect area, twelve children in fact were direct contacts, *yet not a single one in this group developed poliomyelitis.*

There was a second group of sick people—thirty-four in this group, consisting of eighteen white children and sixteen coloured ones. The symptoms varied somewhat, there was muscle tenderness, neck rigidity with temperatures of over a hundred. They were given *Lathyrus Sativus* 30, three doses at half-hourly intervals. The most serious of the cases in this group was a girl of two and a half with neck stiffness and extremely resentful of being touched anywhere. She appeared to be gravely ill, and she was given two doses of *Lathyrus Sativus* 30 half-hourly, after which she fell asleep. By the morning, twelve hours later, the symptoms had disappeared and she was well. Nine cases of the group of thirty-four were seriously ill when seen, and five of them were isolated and nursed at home, but four were sent to hospital for further treatment.

So much for the report by Dr. Taylor Smith on the results of prophylaxis and treatment during a serious epidemic of poliomyelitis treated on Homoeopathic lines; though only a small series, it shows most encouraging results.

There is another factor which should not be overlooked in preparing for an epidemic of this kind, that is the question of fear and anticipation. Many people jump a stile before they ever get there. Fear and panic have a great tendency to lower the morale of a people. Hence the great importance to remain calm and cool in the face of danger. *Gelsemium* is the great remedy for fear and nervous anticipation with trembling and lethargy and will therefore act both as a true prophylactic and a cure in the early days of the onset of the disease.

Suitable vaccines against the disease as a method of protection as in the case of smallpox and yellow fever may be fairly successful, but in my private opinion, Homoeopathy provides an absolutely safe method without any serious after-effects, both for protection and cure of this dreaded disease.

CHOLERA

CHOLERA is one of the most dreaded and most serious epidemic infectious diseases, with an extremely rapid onset and a high mortality rate. Like many other things it has travelled from East to West, hence its name Asiatic cholera. It was reported by travellers as having occurred in the delta of the Ganges by 1629. Nearly 200 years later, in 1827, it spread from Calcutta and China and to Muscat in Arabia, across Asia Minor to the Georgian frontier into Russia, and on from there to Poland and Austria, and gradually it appeared in Hamburg, Germany, and thence to Sunderland in England; always near shipping places and ports. There were various outbreaks in London in the 1830s, and again later the great epidemic of 1854. Always fresh epidemics appeared throughout the next twenty years or more, with high fatalities in its train. For example during Lent 1932, 20,000 people were carried off by it in Paris in one month. It broke out in New York several times about the middle of the century and after.

The mortality of cholera is always around the 50–60 per cent of cases attacked, even now, a hundred years later, the fatality rate is over 40 per cent, nearer 50–55 per cent under prevailing orthodox treatment. How different it is with Homoeopathic treatment, let the following figures tell their own tale.

During an epidemic in New York the death rate under Homoeopathic treatment was 5 per cent. The average death rate of patients treated Homoeopathically both in Europe and America was 9 per cent—both in private and hospital practice.

In Vienna in 1836, the practice of Homoeopathy was forbidden, but cholera was raging so violently in that city that permission was obtained to open an Homoeopathic Cholera Hospital, where the results were so favourable, that two thirds of the patients treated there survived, while two thirds of those treated in other hospitals died. At this startling result, the then Austrian Minister of Interior repealed the law relating to the practice of Homoeopathy in Austria.

In Rheims came the report that of 1,270 patients treated, only 108 died, while the allopathic mortality rate in Russia was between 60–70 per cent. No wonder that after this astounding dénouement of allopathic failure, the Homoeopathic physicians flourished in Russia for several decades. *And* one Homoeopathic doctor in the South of France had a mortality rate of 5–7 per cent while the allopathic death rate in the rest of France was 90 per cent.

Cholera was raging in London in 1854, and twenty-five beds were devoted to the treatment of cholera patients in the London Homoeopathic Hospital, with the satisfying result that only 16 per cent of cases died, while fatality rate of Chelsea under orthodox treatment was 54 per cent. Unfortunately the results have never been published in orthodox medical books. Indeed, one medical body had the following resolution put in its minutes of a meeting that the returns of the results of the Homoeopathic prescribing would give an "unjustifiable sanction to an empirical practice, alike opposed to the maintenance of truth and to the progress of science". Such is the stubbornness of official medicine.

Dr. Rubini had remarkable results in the Naples epidemic of 1854–55. He treated 225 cases of cholera without a single death in Alberge and 166 soldiers of a

Swiss regiment stationed there with the same success. The medicine he found most useful was *"Spirits of Camphor"*.

And this brings me to say a little about the three classic remedies for the treatment of this disease which may break out at any time if there are years of famine and distress.

They are *Camphor, Cuprum* and *Veratrum Alb.*

CAMPHOR symptoms are: extreme icy coldness of the skin, with sudden and absolute prostration of vital force; *face*, livid, purple, icy cold—hippocratic facies, upper lip drawn up exposing the teeth, mouth foaming, eyes sunken and fixed, sudden shrinking of strength and collapse; absent or painless stool. Although the body is icy, the patient will *not* be covered up.

Camphor and collapse are synonymous.

VERATRUM is similar, but there is cold sweat on the forehead and a violent thirst for quantities of ice cold water, and acid drinks. A craving for fruits. Excessive vomiting and purging. As if cold water in the veins.

CUPRUM: Spasmodic, cramping pains. Nausea. Vomiting relieved by drinking cold water. Craves cold drinks. Black painful bloody stools, with weakness and cramp in abdomen. Cramps starting in fingers and toes.

Thus we can summarise these three great remedies for the treatment of cholera—designated by the founder of Homoeopathy—Samuel Hahnemann—and proved through the years by his faithful followers.

CAMPHOR in early stages, when there is collapse, coldness and sudden prostration.

CUPRUM when there is excessive cramps, not only in abdomen, but beginning and continuing in fingers and toes.

VERATRUM ALB.—excessive cold sweat, and excessive vomiting and purging.

TYPHOID

INFECTIOUS or epidemic intestinal disturbances are common, among which are found the enteric groups, the dysenteries, cholera, typhoid and gastric enteritis of the infant, also the so-called food poisoning which is increasing in frequency.

The cause of intestinal upsets, whatever the diagnosis may be is ultimately bound up with lack of cleanliness in preparing food, and lack of care in disposing of human and animal excreta.

The typhoid group of diseases is becoming much less frequent in these islands due to the improved sanitation, and the outbreaks which occur now and then can usually be traced to an unrecognised and mild attack of the disease in an employee on a farm, dairy or any establishment dealing with the handling and preparing of food. Scrupulous cleanliness of the hands and the nails of the cook in the kitchen, the milker on the farm, the shop assistant who handles butter, cheese and processed or fresh meat would reduce the incidence of intestinal infection still further. Also the danger of the ubiquitous fly should be recognised as it settles on decaying material, and later crawls over food. Steps should be taken to cover up all food exhibited in shops, in the kitchen, and the larder.

These dangerous and highly fatal intestinal diseases are mainly found in the East and countries where hygiene is lacking. The importance of public health is rapidly being recognised as vital if life is to be protected, and as time goes on we may see the control and end of these dangerous fevers, including typhoid.

The habits of the people in the Far East are indeed a serious obstacle to the prevention of communicable diseases and are often the breeding place of serious epidemics. In the first week of May, 1951, it was reported in the papers that more than 200 people had died in Calcutta during that week of smallpox, cholera and plague. What an indictment of the lack of warning in public health by the authorities!

The shipping ports all over the world are the greatest points of danger. This is not surprising when you consider that a port is the magnet where the riff-raff of humanity collects; the weak ones and the criminals of the underworld gather here to batten on the unsuspecting sailor, who after weeks of strictest discipline and hard work and the absence of alcohol and female society, has money to burn. He becomes an easy prey to the harpies in the public houses on the dock side, who tempt him with drinks and drugs. He sleeps off his drunken and drugged state in some underground hovel and returns to his ship in due course, often carrying with him the germs of a deadly disease, which may not show for some days or even weeks, when he has landed in another country some thousands of miles away.

When these plague spots of immorality are cleansed, many problems of grave import to the health of communities will be solved.

In considering the Homoeopathic treatment of typhoid, we can divide the fever into three main types —and it will be according to the symptoms found in the individual sufferer that the remedy will be chosen. For the Homoeopathic Law must be followed, that is, it is the individual suffering the disease with the symptoms peculiar to him.

Typhoid fever, at its onset chiefly attacks and modifies the functions of the brain and the digestive organs,

85

and although many cases will be found to be a mixture of symptoms, thereby necessitating the study of each individual case, where there is a preponderance of cerebral symptoms the remedies *Belladonna, Hyoscyamus, Lachesis, Opium* and *Stramonium* should be carefully considered.

The case may begin with the marked symptoms of trembling, with great heaviness and weariness of the limbs, debility, red spots like flea bites or blood stains on the chest, face, neck and abdomen, pain in forehead with excitable delirium, brilliant sparkling eyes in a red face—all of which indicates *Belladonna*, but later after *Belladonna* has been given, these may modify and further symptoms will become apparent. Then to carry the case to its successful conclusion—the drug more closely resembling the modified or changed state will be needed—be it *Arsenicum*, or *Bryonia*, or *Sulphur*.

Typhoid fever may be characterised by predominant abdominal symptoms, and will be met generally by *Arsenicum, Carbo. Veg, China, Colchicum, Mercurius, Nux Moschata, Secale* and *Sulphur*.

The third variety of typhoid is that in which the cerebral and abdominal symptoms are both present, neither of which can be said to predominate. Here *Bryonia* will play an important part, but any case may need *Arnica, Calcarea, Nux Vomica, Pulsatilla, Rhus Tox*, or *Veratrum A*.

Every case will be different, and the cure which can be made by Homoeopathy, will depend always on the care which is taken, at the bedside of the patient, to observe and note every detail which will be characteristic and peculiar to him. Care taken in the early stages will ensure good results and a happy deliverance from what can be a serious and fatal disease, coupled always with the strict observance of cleanliness at all times—particularly in the handling and protection of food.

TYPHUS

First let me make it quite clear that typhus is not the same as typhoid. Typhoid or enteric is a disease of the small intestine, generally associated with the typhoid bacillus—while typhus is a disease affecting the cerebral organ, the brain. It is a brain fever, not an abdominal or bowel condition. Until the days when the improvement of the microscope led to the study of bacteriology, the two diseases were often mistaken one for the other; but typhus is by far the more serious of the two; that is judging from the high death rate of typhus.

The health authorities in this country are getting anxious about typhus; it is creeping closer and closer. The accompaniment and repercussions of war and famine and pestilence, and the dread horsemen of the Apocalypse are now riding over the war scarred plains of Europe, famine first and then comes pestilence stalking in its wake—in other words typhus.

It is called colloquially by other names, such as camp fever, ship fever or jail fever. It is associated with overcrowded places, camps, etc. In one camp recently, in Greece, a correspondent writes in a few terse sentences —"and then typhus struck one camp and out of 300 prisoners only twenty to thirty survived", and he amongst them—so 90 per cent of the camp died from typhus. Another camp, in the South of France, where the sanitary arrangements were indescribable, was attacked by typhus, and again the death rate was just on 90 per cent. In both these camps there was then no medical aid available; but in another camp a highly qualified British medical man was among the prisoners of war, and he struggled hard to overcome the enemy, but in spite of everything he succumbed as well to this disease. No wonder typhus is dreaded.

An acquaintance of mine who knew a Russian lady who had experienced a typhus epidemic, her comment was "well, whoever was attacked by typhus, just died, nothing could be done for them". In 1936—46,000 cases of typhus occurred in Ethiopia, Russia and in Spain. Four thousand five hundred cases were reported during the first months of 1941, and nearly 1,200 cases during the same period in 1941 in Germany.

Rumour has it that typhus is raging in Greece and the Balkan states, and the mortality rate is said to be appalling.

Typhus was also known as ship fever. This was common in the days when the Negroes were forcibly abducted from their homes in Africa and thrown in their hundreds into the holds of the ships which took them over to America to serve as slaves in the sugar plantations. Overcrowded and starved, they died off like flies before they ever arrived in America.

Jail fever, another name for typhus, was caused by the appalling conditions in which the prisoners were kept in the jails; specially the debtors' prisons; dirty, filthy; no facilities for cleanliness; huddled together in crowds, defective sanitation, poor food; sooner or later typhus or jail fever made its appearance. In order to protect the judges and barristers against the infection from the dangerous diseases rife in the prisoners, it was the custom to strew aromatic herbs, hyssop, rosemary, about the court. You will perhaps recall that Charles Dickens wrote his novel *Little Dorrit* in order to show up the awful conditions which existed in the debtors' prison at the Marshalsea—which has since been pulled down; but the name is still kept alive, in the Marshalsea Buildings in Southwark, near London Bridge.

This was barely one hundred years ago. We do not realise how much we have done to improve social conditions all round in a few decades. Up to 1869 jail fever or typhus was prevalent in Britain and some 6,000–8,000 people died of it every year. Various laws were passed then, and the water boards were formed for supplying a pure water supply. Then the Public Health Acts of 1875 made the provision of drains and sewers compulsory. A clean water supply, proper drainage and sewage system—good hygiene all round—had the desired effects at once. Typhus disappeared, and for seventy years there has been no return in Britain, thus clearly proving that typhus was due to faulty hygiene; merely a dirt and filth disease; a disease easily controlled by cleanliness. Clean fresh water and soap will abolish dirt, and will reduce fleas and lice which love to dwell in dirt.

It has been discovered, a little over twenty years ago, that typhus can be passed on from one person to another by means of carrier lice. Certain cells were found, and called after the Russian scientist who first spotted them, Rickettsiae prowazekii. There were plenty of opportunities to study typhus in Poland and Russia where this disease is endemic. I knew people who used to travel in Russia in the 1930s and used to complain bitterly of the unwelcome visitors they picked up in the trains.

The public health authorities everywhere are tightening up their preventive measures. They go all out for prevention. It is essential it is stated, to have a large number of personnel who are thoroughly trained in carrying out the cleansing of human beings and their property, or as it is put baldly in official language "The delousing of people". The sanitary personnel must be well trained in the methods, they are supplied with voluminous overalls which cover them all over, hands and feet are firmly tied in, a hood is drawn over the head, they wear gloves and special boots, so that each member is well protected against a stray visitor. They indeed look more like representatives of a secret Ku-Klux Klan than staid British sanitary officials. Disinfecting bunkers are provided, where clothes, blankets, bedding, can be disinfected; and the people themselves are bathed and their lice got rid of.

To prevent lice carrying the disease from Poland into Germany, the regulation has been made that anyone crossing the frontier from east to west, both soldiers and civilians, must undergo a triple delousing process. Everywhere on the Continent lice are increasing in an alarming manner, but this is not surprising if you consider that fats and soap and coal are at a premium. Household fuel is difficult to obtain so that washing facilities are difficult. Furthermore, where malnutrition is present in the population, as under war conditions, when it is difficult to provide sufficient protective food, milk, butter, eggs, in order to keep up a high standard of health, and it strains the available economics and food resources of the civil authorities to provide enough fuel, soap, water and food for everybody, the result is inevitable—lice can increase.

The modern health authorities would prefer it, if a suitable cheap method of vaccination could be evolved, which would prevent the disease. Attempts have been made to prepare a vaccine which would safely and effectively immunise against typhus ever since the Rickettsiae lice have been recognised as the causative agents. They have made preparations from fleas and lice, disgusting mixtures, which have been injected into human beings, as preventives. For example, a living typhus virus was injected into 500 people in an asylum in Europe, but it only caused a severe reaction and the mortality rate and the number attacked was uninfluenced by it. In fact it has been found that such a vaccine made from living lice increased the severity of the epidemic.

Then another vaccine was made by adding carbolic acid to the intestinal contents of lice infected with the Rickettsiae obtained from the brains of infected guinea pigs. This method necessitated a huge stock of lice, which in this form could only be kept alive by feeding on immune persons, that is the laboratory staff. So an extra large staff of persons had to be supplied to keep the lice—and from 200–300 lice were necessary for one person—so this method was impossible for the preparation of vaccine for large scale immunisation.

The latest vaccine which has been evolved is from the findings of Cox. He found that the Rickettsii grew profusely in the yolk sacs of developing chick embryos. You get enough vaccine for twenty-five to thirty people from fourteen chick embryos—a disgusting method, and one still asks—is it of sufficient value, does it really protect against typhus?

These vaccines of killed Rickettsii have been found to protect experimental animals against the disease in the laboratories, but the results are not so satisfactory in man.

Some of the laboratory staff who submitted to the vaccine treatment were infected with typhus even though they had three or more vaccine injections sufficiently long beforehand for the immune anti-bodies to develop. The Americans, the Rockefellers workers inoculated some 20,000 people in Spain with the serum in 1941—but were forced to leave Spain, before they could get any data, whether the vaccination was effective or not.

Not one of the medical authorities either in America

or England can say whether their vaccines, however disgusting their method of preparations are, are of any use in protecting the individual for certain against an attack of typhus; and in Russia and Germany they are not allowed to carry out large scale immunisations with vaccines the sources of which are unknown, or where methods and results are also unknown, i.e. unproven.

In America and Great Britain, the amount of vaccine available is insufficient (fortunately perhaps) to start a campaign for general immunisation for everybody. There is more or less compulsory immunising of the delousing and sanitary staffs. They are warned that they are running risks, that the results are uncertain, but still for the country's sake, etc., they should be willing to run the risk and allow themselves to be vaccinated.

I have already in my lecture on diphtheria immunisation, tried to point out that there are dangers and risks attendant on the multiplication of serum inoculations for protection against each and every infectious disease. The danger of anaphylaxis, serum shock and sudden death is always present in these cases. The danger is very great and largely due to phenomena which the lay people and even the ordinary medical practitioner who remembers little about electricity or physics, does not fully appreciate. The danger is that the radiations which are emitted by every living being, are being upset by others of different values and vibration.

Life is the outcome of radiation and vibration, taking place in the nuclei, the centre of each cell. Without this radiation there would be no life. Natural radiation is essential for life and as soon as the nucleus is destroyed, vibration or oscillation in it ceases and the cell dies. Now, it has been proved by experiments that the vital cells in the human body emit electrons generated by an actual radio-activity whose intensity is much greater than that observed in animals and plants.

And the microbe or bacteria is a living organism, just another cell which vibrates with a frequency differing from that of the organic human cell; therefore if bacteria enters the human body, a disharmony will be caused within it, and the electrical equilibrium will be disturbed. The human cell is thus forced to vibrate under abnormal conditions, and because the cell does not function normally it becomes diseased. The microbes are cells containing a nucleus, and emit radiations, and when these elementary forms of life come into contact with the highly organised human cells, there is a war of radiation between healthy cells and microbes. This is a problem analagous to the difficulty a person finds himself in who works to rescue his friend who is in danger. He faces powerful aggressors, but dare not make use of his weapons for fear of endangering his friend who is struggling with the enemy. Similarly it is difficult to destroy the microbe without destroying the living cells of the human body.

It has been proved that every cell oscillates with a frequency and wave length which is determined by the size of its particular filaments. And therefore by virtue of the form and size of the filament, every cell, like every microbe possesses its own wave length characteristic of its species. And if we modify the make-up of the filaments as its conductive capacity, by chemical means or by injections, other cells of a different electro-magnetic make-up, we modify the frequency of the vibration; and we modify the particular character of the cell and produce an alteration in it. We may age it prematurely, or it may become deformed, diseased or transmuted in some way. Therefore introducing disease products such as dead bacteria or serums from a body, from other animals, into the organic cells of the human body is reprehensible and should be strongly deprecated. Latent disease of the filaments of cells is caused which may take months or years to develop and seriously disturb the harmony of the body.

The allopathic school can only offer you very doubtful means of combating typhus—what can Homoeopathy offer?

In 1813 there was a war on the Continent. The war had lasted for seven years and more, food was scarce, and typhus developed. It was treated by Hahnemann according to the Homoeopathic Law—that like cures like. He found a certain combination of symptoms in the cases he saw which in the first stage of the disease corresponded to either *Bryonia* or *Rhus Tox*; and in the second stage of the disease, resembled the action of *Hyoscyamus* which he gave in the 12th centesimal dilution. Hahnemann saw and treated 183 patients and this treatment was so effective that all of them recovered. Hahnemann was an idealist and wanted to shout the news from the housetops, that typhus could be cured. So he published his cases and the particulars of his treatment with the minutest details, in the best-known papers of that day, not looking for any rewards for himself, he wished to save future victims. What was the result?—he was maligned, jeered at and completely ostracised. Other medical professors made his life unbearable, nothing but jealousy and bias, because they could not cure typhus, they declared it was incurable; whoever said it was curable, was a liar.

It is 130 years ago since Hahnemann performed his miracle and cured all his cases of typhus. Homoeopathy is still being taught, it still lives, and it can and will do the same. It will cure cases of typhus, but there are no specifics, even for typhus. Each case must be observed individually; all details must be watched, observed and noted down and then the particular type of the prevailing epidemic will be found and cures will take place as before.

The natural law, the law of similars, still holds good. If faced with an epidemic of typhus, the procedure would be the same. Ignore the name of the disease. Carefully watch each person attacked; write down all the little symptoms, the behaviour of the patient whether restless or not, whether stupid, sleepy, comatose or delirious; the character of the muttering—whether intelligible or not; some patients are excitable in their delirium, others are depressed, mutter and jabber, or are wildly stupidly delirious. Some are difficult to nurse; some recognise their relatives and attendants. According to the best ensemble of the symptoms of the patient—you would have to find corresponding to him, the similar remedy—not an easy matter. It may be *Arsenicum*, it may be *Hyoscyamus*, it may be *Bryonia* or *Rhus Tox*. Never become a routinist and work according to rule of thumb. Because *Bryonia* and *Rhus Tox*. cured all the cases in Hahnemann's day it does not mean they will cure the cases in the future. Each epidemic has its own symptoms, needs its particular drug to cure. Do not give *Aconite* because there is fever present. *Aconite* is not a remedy for continuous fever. *Belladonna, Hyoscyamus, Lachesis, Opium, Stramonium*, may be needed for the delirium. *Arsenicum* may be needed in those cases where there is anxiety and restlessness, prostration and weepiness; but never in a comatose state. If in high fever there is thirstlessness, remember *Pulsatilla*, but if there is a dry mouth, the tongue sticks to the roof of the mouth, distention of the abdomen with much flatulence, great sleepiness and giddiness as of drink, stupid delirium, remember *Nux Moschata*—the nutmeg. *Pulsatilla, Sulphur, Secale, Mercury, Arnica, Lycopodium*, you may need in fact any one remedy.

The only way is to find out is to study each individual patient as I have said before; if there is an epidemic and many people are attacked it will be easier, for the great majority will then show the same symptoms; and any particular epidemic responds as a rule to two or three remedies.

Personally, I have no fear of typhus for I doubt whether it will ever reach these shores. If we had to live in underground caves without water or soap, crowded together, typhus could break out. A clean, reasonably fed nation need not be afraid of typhus. Only a dirty nation, forced underground, overcrowded, short of soap and cleaning materials, reduced by lack of food and clean water need fear this disease. God forbid that such things should ever happen here, but if they did, the treatment still would be—right the conditions and use the remedies indicated by the application of the Homoeopathic Law of Similars.

INDEX